Diet Well

Diet Well

Healthy Lifestyle Leads to Happy Life

Authored by

SONIA KOCHAR

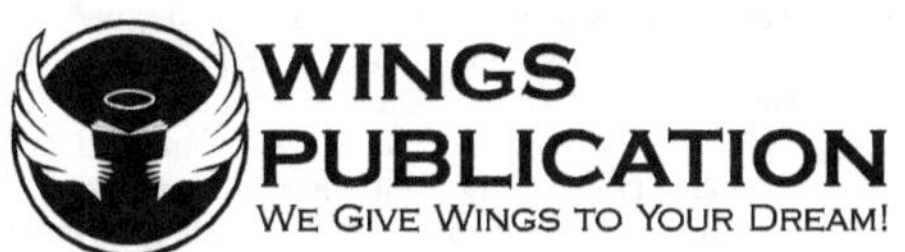

Disclaimer

This book has been published with all reasonable efforts taken to make the material error-free after the consent of the author. This book is sold subject to the condition that it shall not, by way of trade or otherwise, be lent, resold, or otherwise circulated without the copyright owner's prior written consent in any form of binding or cover other than that in which it is published and without a similar condition including this condition being imposed on the subsequent purchaser and without limiting the rights under copyright reserved above, no part of this publication maybe reproduced, stored in or introduced into a retrieval system or transmitted in any form or by any other means without the permission of the copyright owner.

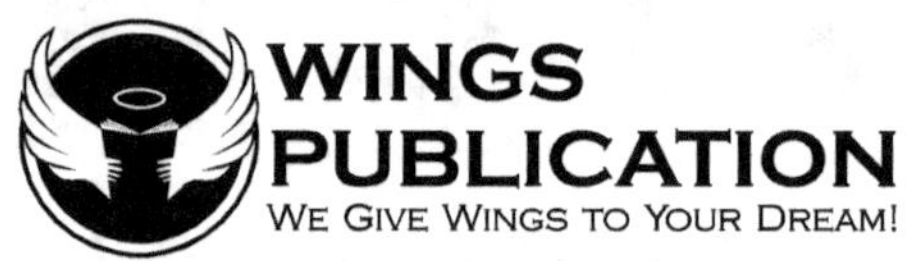

Registered Office- 907-Sneh Nagar, Sapna Sangeeta Road, Agrasen Square, Indore – 452001 (M.P.), India
Website: http://www.wingspublication.com
Email: mybook@wingspublication.com

First Published by WINGS PUBLICATION 2020
Copyright © SONIA KOCHAR 2020

Title: Diet Well
Price: ₹499 / $10
All Rights Reserved.
ISBN 978-81-947142-7-9

LIMITS OF LIABILITY/DISCLAIMER OF WARRANTY

Dedication

I would like to dedicate this wonderful book of mine to my parents, for being the pillars of my strength, constant source of inspiration and guidance – Almighty God for planting the seed of this creation in me, through his will, for his never-ending blessings and miracles in my life.

This is a Miracle too.

Acknowledgements

Besides our family, throughout our life, we meet many people, who stroll this curious journey of life alongside us. Some, only a few steps while others stay and walk all the way with us. I have been fortunate enough to have a handful of such people in my life. Though we don't get a lot of chances to give them their due credit or as is human's profound defect, take them for granted. But now as this book, which is no less than a part of me as well as a new beginning makes its way into the world, I'd like to tell those people how much they mean to me and how thankful I am, for their presence.

- *All those super-heroes including nutritionists, diet-professionals, healers, trainers who are working or have worked and dedicated their whole lives towards making people fitter each day, and making this world a better place for them. You might know this, or not, but you are making significant contribution to their happiness, making them sleep peacefully at night and increasing the span of their lives as well. Cheers to you guys!*

- *All the people I have worked with, the world calls them clients, but they're like my extended family. Every time they gain a pound, I get uneasy and their depressions leads to frown and creases on my forehead. I want to tell them that they have made me really proud and each of their successes is a shiny new feather to my hat. I hope and pray that all of you will keep moving forward like this.*

- *And of course, how can I forget my dedicated and loyal readers? They are my inspiration and my reason to write. And I'd be really satisfied and ecstatic if I can help the readers in any way, whether nutritionally and spiritually. Also, I am eternally grateful to everyone who took precious moments from such hectic and a life that is on the move all the time to read what I have penned down.*

- *I would like to thank my whole family, my super supportive husband and my kids for being the constant pillars of support, for putting up with all my moods during the writing sessions and the grumpiness of the writers' block. None of this would have been possible without the three of you. Trust me, not a page!*

- *A customary thanks to the almighty whose will we all follow and I have been fortunate enough to come out with something so special owing to his will. I am grateful and I feel blessed to be an object of his worthy direction, in not only writing this book, but in each and every sphere of this wonderful life he has bestowed upon me.*

In the end, I'd like to motivate my readers to give healthy way of life a fair try. I promise the way it'll make you feel will have you never turning back towards the sluggish junk-eating lifestyle ever again. But quitting won't work. Give it a good 2-3 months to see and feel the difference in you.

Happy Reading!

Preface

When it's the question of introducing the book, how do you introduce something that is the amalgamation of your go-to nutritionist , with no need to take appointments and who could be by your side 24/7, a spiritual mentor to take away all your self-doubts, who helps you see the light at the end of the tunnel and provides the peace and serenity we all keep looking for throughout our lives, but never find it, and a provider of scientifically correct information rather than some blah **Myth**s to misguide you? I'd leave all that to you, dear Reader.

Moving on, I think it's pretty obvious why I chose to write this book. Apart from the fact that nutrition is my passion and profession, and helping people out a long striven-for goal, let us just acknowledge and affect the fact that weight problems are becoming more and more prominent and ominous nowadays. Walk out of your houses, stroll around the balcony for a few moments and it is very unlikely to find someone who is not overweight. In fact, you could even overhear someone cribbing about their weight to their best friend and fretting over that gooey dessert they could not resist at the party last evening and how the calorie count spiked up and they're feeling all guilty.

I mean really, it is everyone's story. 90% or more of the people want to lose weight, get that perfect figure, abs or a flat stomach, but a bigger part of this population does not or cannot work towards achieving that. The reasons are not that varying. The same story, someone can't get desserts out of their mind, while the other loves their stuffed bread with a dollop of homemade butter on the top and pickles on the side. That, my friend, makes dieting a hard nut to crack for most people.

The book provides the necessary guidance equipped with scientifically proven facts to all those who are willing to brush their favourite foods aside till the weekend, follow health regime all week, exercise regularly, think positively and indulge carefully on the weekends. It can be your best friend if you follow everything it says religiously. I mean it.

Furthermore, to promote good health and well-being in the society, I have started a new concept.

I am the organiser of 'Diet Well Health Awareness Club' for ladies in which we take care of women health issues which we generally neglect in taking care of families. So, we have special coffee sessions where we invite gynaecologist, dermatologists, and oncologists to discuss on various aspects of women healthcare. We make sure that the members of the club get their 'full body profile tests' done and come to know about their bodies well. Mammography and Pap smear tests are also in this package.

Apart from women healthcare, we are into social work too. We often visit orphanages, old age homes, and slum areas to help poor and needy people. We have various workshops with motivational speakers, spiritual healers who guide women to look forward in their lives.

It is a real good combination of physical, mental, and social well-being.

Now is the part when we discuss a serious and unfortunate issue that makes us a little less proud and a little more worried about our country. The issue, although, is not new, has not been considered under the spot light, not at least till the advent on the controversial yet the on-point concept of feminism. Those who still can't get it, I am talking about the grave mistake people do of associating weight with beauty. Yes, I am all up for willing to make yourself better, but listen to me when I say this:

YOU ARE NOT UGLY IF YOU ARE FAT

Do not let anybody tell you otherwise. Each one of us in perfect in a very unique way. Do not let those nosy relatives get under your skin when they tell you that nobody is going to marry you if you don't shed the belly fat.

This book guides you on these lines, motivates you to love yourself and do right by yourself. Because self-love is the best kind of love.

If we talk about men, especially those who are into high-end life-saving professions, its mostly the fact that they are always on clock and they don't have moments to grab that much-needed breakfast, a healthy lunch and a well-balanced dinner, so the only option left to them to keep themselves full is grabbing that mayonnaise laden sandwich and the over sweet coffee from the canteen. Calories mostly take a back-seat in these situations.

And when we talk about our ambitious lovely ladies, balancing their homes, their jobs and their toddlers, the basic instinct is to be blamed. Which undoubtedly is the one of putting every one ahead of her. She takes everyone to the doctor but takes her own weight casually. Not that her family does not appreciate the efforts, they do, but won't it make them happier of the ladies could take just a little time for themselves? Definitely.

So, what is needed in both these cases, is a customized yet general diet, making you understand all the good and bad effect, each article you eat, has on your body. Also, a major amount of stress is upon losing weight without having to starve yourself, following all the right techniques.

Last but not the least, It guides you, and deals with all the issues like depression, anxiety, stress, worries and everything else under the mental health umbrella and aims at curing it all, healing you spiritually and leading you towards the life you always wished for.

People are often unreasonable, Illogical and self-centred
Forgive them anyway.

* * *

If you are kind, people may accuse you of selfish motives.
Be kind anyway.

* * *

If you are successful, you will earn some false friends
and some true friends.
Succeed Anyway.

* * *

If you spend years building, someone could destroy
overnight. Build anyway.

* * *

If you find serenity and Peace, they may be jealous
Be happy anyway.

* * *

The good you do today, people will often forget
tomorrow. Do good anyway.

* * *

Give the world the best you have and
it may never be enough
Give them your best anyway.

* * *

In the final analysis, it is between you and God.
It was never between you and them anyway.

* * *

Contents

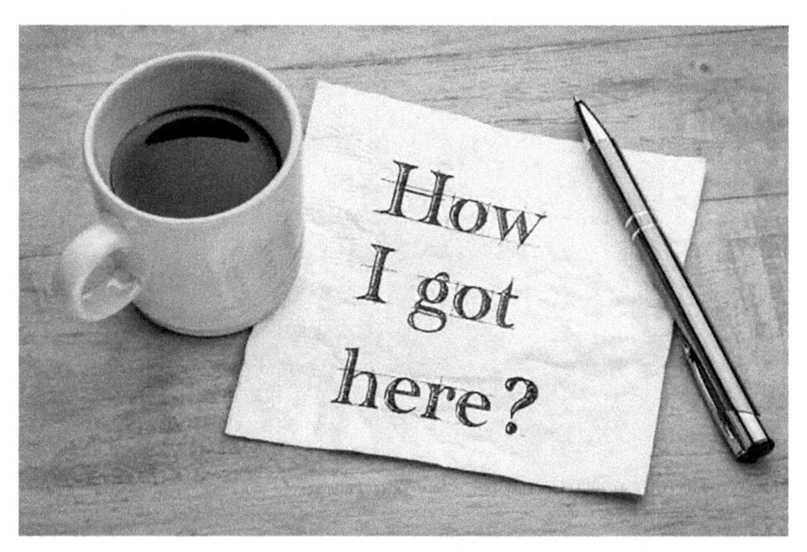

CHAPTER

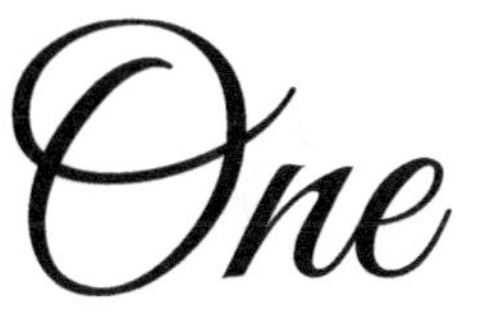

Discipline Is the Key to Success

'For every disciplined effort, there is a multiple reward'
– Jim Rohn

When you think of the word discipline you may be thinking of being scolded by a teacher or a parent or think of the rigid procedures followed by the military. Discipline does not sound like fun. Those who see, learn, and grow, see discipline quite differently. They recognize is that true discipline is truly an ally, a vehicle that allows you to achieve the results you want to attain.

People associate diet or healthy eating with deprivation of food and giving up all the pleasures. If you also think the same, change the concept in your mind.

Start associating self-discipline with inner strength and courage and not with giving into harmful eating habits and laziness. This still can help you gain more control over your life, your actions, and your reactions.

Why self-discipline is good for your health?

1. It helps you to stop eating unhealthy food:

Eating too much food, eating junk and eating too much sugar are not good for health. A great number of people have no control over their eating habits due to lack of discipline and lack of inner strength. If they had some discipline they could reduce the quantity of food they eat, avoid junk food, and consume less sugar.

Discipline would help us eat in a more healthy way.

2. It helps you reduce the amount of alcohol you drink

When you possess a disciplined life, it becomes easier to reduce the amount of alcohol you drink. Having 1-2 drinks is ok for most people. However, when we overindulge in this, it is a bad habit and, may create problems in our lives.

Possessing self-discipline can help you resist drinking and the temptation to drink too much.

3. It enables you to exercise properly

Nowadays, we all avoid physical activities and prefer to slouch on the couch, watch TV, or be on our laptops, mobiles and eat junk food when we're at home. If we developed even a small degree of self-discipline, we would be able to make ourselves go to the gym, walk, or do any other exercise.

Exercising is essential for our health. When you have discipline you do not succumb to laziness and procrastination. It gives you the strength to get out of bed and do the exercises you love.

4. It helps you lose weight

Many people come to me, who have been trying to lose weight but end up breaking their own resolve due to a lack of self-discipline. They can't resist the tasty food and ice-creams. Do you realize what is stopping you from losing weight? It is only a lack of self-confidence and discipline.

Just imagine how slim could be, if you have control over the foods you eat or if you could say 'no' to bad foods.

I promise it is not that difficult, but the thing is when you want to start. Follow disciplined habits of early dinner eating, healthy eating, and saying 'no' to the junk food, hydrate yourself properly and you are very much near the right and desired weight.

5. It enables you to control anger

Anger is not good for health. It affects our minds and bodies adversely. It increases your blood pressure. You need to restrain your anger, resist being dragged into unnecessary arguments, and avoid raising your voice.

To be able to do so, you do self-discipline and inner strength.

6. It helps you overcome all the unhealthy habits

Smoking, overeating, eating junk food and unhealthy food, laziness, procrastination, or other negative habits harm your health. However, you can overcome these habits and build positive habits if you possess the skill of self-discipline.

In order to live a better and healthy life and have better control over your actions, you need to sustain a degree of self-control. Its possession enables you to resist temptations and distractions, improve endurance, and help you overcome negative habits.

Simple Changes in Life to Reach Your Goal

Self-discipline requires practice and repetition in your day-to-day life. To improve your self-discipline test out these 5 proven methods to gain better control.

This regime will help you to improve your control by making simple changes to your everyday routine.

1. Remove temptations

Self-control is often the easiest when abiding by the saying: 'Out of sight, out of mind'

Removing all the temptations and distractions is the crucial first step when working to improve your self-discipline. If you are trying to control your eating, toss the junk food out. If you want to improve your focus while working, switch off your cell phone, and remove the clutter from your desk. Set yourself up for success by ditching the bad influences.

2. Eat Regularly and healthily

We need to focus on our health. When you are hungry, your ability to concentrate suffers as your brain is no functioning to its highest potential.

Hunger makes it difficult to focus on the tasks in hand, making you grumpy and pessimist. You have less control over your life, diet, work, relationships. In order to stay on track, make sure that you are well-fuelled throughout the day, with healthy snacks and meals, every few hours.

These snacks ensure than you get a healthy dose of protein and fat throughout the day when needed. Eating often regulates our blood sugar level and improves our decisions making skills and concentration.

3. Don't wait for it to feel right

Improving your self-discipline means changing your normal routine, which can be uncomfortable and awkward. When our behaviour becomes a habit, we stop using our decision-making skills and instead function on auto-pilot mode. Therefore breaking bad habits and making new habits not only requires us making active decisions, but it will also feel wrong. Your brain will resist the change in favour of what it has been programmed to do.

Acknowledge that it will take a while for your new regime to feel right or good or natural. Keep changing along. It will happen soon.

4. Schedule breaks, treats, and rewards for yourself

While practicing self-discipline, schedule specific breaks, treats and rewards for yourself. Dieting? Designate Saturdays as ice-cream sundae day. Schedule the treats. Have ice-cream in the noon or at 4 pm and balance your evening and dinner time (light meal). Self-discipline can be hard, reward your efforts. Pat yourself on the back if you balance the healthy eating and the rewards well.

5. Forgive yourself and move forward

Instituting a new way of thinking won't always go according to the plan. You will have ups and downs, fabulous successes, and flat-out failures. The key is to keep moving forward. When you have a setback, acknowledge what caused it and move on. It is easy to get wrapped in guilt, anger, or frustration. Forgive yourself and get back in the saddle ASAP. It is better to forgive yourself and move forward in a positive direction.

"Discipline is the foundation of a positive and a happy life."

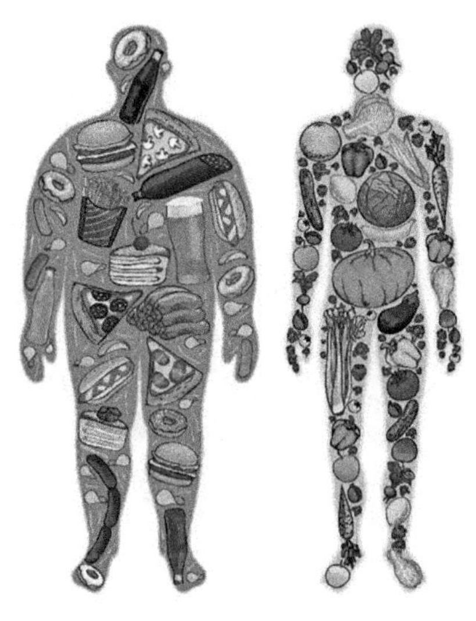

CHAPTER

Two

Healthy Weight Loss

Are you overweight?

90% population of India or I can say Punjab is struggling with weight issues today. I can't see a house in my colony or any of my friends who are not struggling with the same. The main reason for weight gain is we are getting increasingly addicted to electronic gadgets, spend hours watching TV, working or playing games on the computer, tweeting with Friends, checking and updating our Facebook profiles, texting on our phones, and searching to get solutions to our life's issues.

A few decades back, when we were younger, we would spend our days playing with friends, walk in the park but now we're always indoors. All of these habits make us lazy and sedentary and as a result, we put on weight. We also have easy access to junk, instant, and fried foods. They are the answer to our hunger pangs. But we don't realize that they're fattening and difficult to digest.

When a 26-year-old girl came to me to lose weight, she was 69kgs at that moment. The main reason for weight gain was late-night binge eating. Most of the youth have this weakness. They are awake at night using gadgets, binge eating chips, chocolates, donuts, colas, etc. which are their favourite late-night meals. My client had a sweet tooth problem. She loved eating sweets, ice-creams, and brownies. Although she was trying to control her weight, instead of coming down, it was spiralling upwards. She had started experiencing sharp mood swings and getting irritated at trivial things.

I started counselling her and ask her to leave one weakness at a time. We decided to start with sweets. In her first week, without sweets, she lost 3 kgs. This was the time, she got motivated to lose more weight.

Slowly, steadily, she had control over her weakness and lost 12kgs in 3 months. She started meditating and looking at the positive aspects of life and today she has completely accepted a healthy lifestyle.

This is the journey we can guide you on but in the end, you have to have good self-control and adapt a healthy lifestyle and stick to it for the rest of your life.

Now, she is a completely transformed personality. She is slim and smiling and looks a lot younger than she used to when I first saw her.

Difference between Overweight and Obese

How are overweight and obese different? When you consume more calories than you can burn out, you start accumulating the excess calories in your body as fat. That fat gets deposited as a layer under your skin. You are overweight when you cross the threshold of ideal body weight.

Obesity is the advanced stage of being overweight and actually a disease, which can lead to serious medical conditions like high blood pressure and other heart diseases, diabetes, osteoporosis, digestive problems, sleep disorders, backache, and many more. Interestingly, fat or adipose tissues are formed in most of us in our childhood. And once these tissues are formed they keep troubling us intermittently. We all adore plump babies but we are harming them by overfeeding them and making them lethargic and dull.

There are many reasons for putting up weight, but the most common ones are wrong eating habits, overeating, and leading a sedentary lifestyle. We don't get much time to exercise due to a heavy workload, which leaves us feeling exhausted by the end of the day.

Some have a complete lack of motivation to lose weight. Some feel as they don't have to face cameras, it does not matter much. Most commonly, people love to eat whatsoever comes in front of them. They don't really mind putting on some extra kgs on their body and go out of shape. They have short-lived targets. They would like to lose weight if a family wedding is approaching. They would do any diet, fasting, crash diet, a keto diet, net searching, and in the end would land up where they started their journey.

When you are overweight you have an opportunity of losing weight much sooner than the obese category. In fact, in some cases, you can get back to your ideal weight with very few alterations in your daily routine, correcting diet, 30 minutes work out, and leaving a sedentary lifestyle. However, when you are obese it takes more time, effort, dedication, and discipline to get back into shape.

Motivation is the Key

Motivation is near you, within you- but you just can't see it. Just like we make time for eating, sleeping, and electronic gadgets, which we think are important, the same way we can find time for exercise. Taking care of your body is very important. So start loving your body. Get some free time from your busy schedules and exercise. Focus on your well-being.

There are also others who think they don't need to lose weight. They think they are too fat or too old to lose weight. They hate to look at themselves in the mirror and avoid ever going near weighing scales. In short, they have totally given up hope. They too want to lose weight but think it is not possible anymore. I want to tell you all that 'you can'.

I had a client, a 22-year-old boy who was 120kgs when he came to me. He felt it was an impossible task to lose weight as he had a sedentary lifestyle, working on the laptop who night and sleeping the whole day. Slowly, steadily, after 2-3 counselling sessions, he tried to set his working hours and eating habits. Slowly his sleeping patterns were set and his life completely changed. Within 3 months, he lost 21kgs and left junk food, and scheduled his day according to me.

Then he hardly visited me, and now he has a perfect weight. Today, he is 95kgs and he is a very happy guy.

You too can embrace good health and lose weight. You just need counselling and the right motivation. Just take

80-90 minutes out of your busy schedules, because you owe that to yourself and your body.

Good health is for everybody.

Know Your Ideal Weight

Ideal body weight is the most important marker of fitness. It is your weight as per your age, gender, height, body structure. It is different for different people. Any excess weight applies stress on your joints and back, causes health problems like high cholesterol, heart blockage, and diabetes, etc.

Balanced weight and height of a particular body structure is must and can be achieved through a healthy diet, physical training, and mental balance. Getting to know your ideal weight is like the first step towards fitness. The next step is to figure out how much of the extra pounds that you've piled on you need to lose. Then start working hard towards losing weight earnestly.

We all have different body types. Some of us are small-framed while others have large or medium frames. You can find out your ideal body weight with the help of an expert. An easy way to check your ideal weight is to calculate your BMI (Body Mass Index).

It is a person's weight in kg divided by the square of height in meters. A high BMI can be an indicator of high body fatness. BMI is a convenient rule of thumb used to broadly categorize a person as underweight, normal weight, overweight or obese, based on the tissue mass and height.

The commonly accepted BMI ranges are underweight (under 18.8 kg/m²), normal weight (18.5-25), overweight (25-30), and obese (over 30).

Deal with Water Retention

Water retention is the main cause of weight gain. I know many women who say 'Even though I eat healthily and exercise daily, I am still not able to lose weight'. They feel so frustrated. It happens due to water retention in their bodies.

A simple test to see if you have water retained in your body is to press the skin of your thighs and arm if the skin wrinkles after you pinch it, you have water retention.

Now, how to deal with it?

Most people would start drinking an even lesser amount of water, not knowing that water deficiency is the main cause of water retention. So the less water you drink the more water will get accumulated in your body. If we drink less water our kidneys can't filter out all the toxins from the body. These toxins get stored in the muscles making them weak and flabby.

One of the reasons for water retention is the intake of excess salt. Our bodies need 2-3 grams of salt each day for normal functioning. Canned or tinned foods, salad dressings, packaged foods, soups, curries, etc. have excess salts and should be avoided. In fact, replace normal salt with rock salt in your food.

- Don't add extra salt in salads and fruits.
- Spinach, mushrooms, cabbage don't need extra salt

and can be cooked with very little or no salt.

- Never have rice for dinner, it makes you feel heavy and turns into water during the night.
- Have salt less omelette and nimbu paani.

How to Cure Water Retention

Drink more water to cure water retention. Drink at least 4-5 litres of water in a day. Try to store water in copper vessels and drink it in silver glasses for good digestion, which in turn reduces water retention and weight gain. Drink water at regular intervals throughout the day.

Water for Life

The role of water in our bodies is vital and complex and helps in regulating weight and living well.

- Water is essential for the fat-burning process. If you are dehydrated your metabolism slows down and you will not burn fat fast.
- Water flushes out all toxins, which are produced by an active metabolism and high BMR.
- Water prevents acidity and dilutes the contents of the stomach.
- If you increase the amount of fibre in the diet, you need extra water to help fibre to pass out of your body as waste.
- Dehydration causes a domino effect when your blood volume reduces due to inadequate water, your muscles will suffer from cramps and a feeling of tiredness.
- Water is also known to prevent migraines.

- Drink lukewarm water or water at room temperature for the best results.
- To keep your body running smoothly and skin glowing, you must drink 3-4 liters of water a day.

Right Ways to Drink Water

- Start your day with 2 glasses of lukewarm lemon water.
- Carry a water bottle with you wherever you go.
- Drink water in the form of soups, lemon water, coconut water, green tea, green coffee, and juices.
- Measure out the amount of water you need to drink and keep drinking throughout the day until you have drunk it all.
- Too much water is dangerous as it will dilute the amount of sodium in your body.
- Spread your water intake throughout the day and do not consume the recommended amount all at once.

10 Steps for Weight Management

If your skin looks dry and flaky, the chances are you are not drinking enough water. A well-hydrated skin glows and is firm to touch. You need to change your life holistically with healthy eating, exercise, and relaxation regime.

1. **Eat right** – Eat foods that are essential for good health and active metabolism foods that are rich in fibre, protein, and minerals.
2. **Eat Often** – You need to eat three main meals and 4-6 small meals a day, including healthy snacks, fruits, and vegetables.

3. **Eat Just Enough** – Size matters a lot, so try to eat small portions of food in the right combinations. Focus on portion sizes which will help you regulate your diet.

4. **Drink plenty of water and beverages** – To hydrate, detoxify and nourish your system, drink at least 3 litres of water a day, in addition to anti-oxidants and detoxifying beverages like vegetable juices, green tea, and nutrient-rich coconut water.

5. **Pamper your taste buds** – You need to eat tasty and healthy foods. We need to indulge in our favourite foods with a healthy twist, of course. Try healthy recipes and eat your favourite foods.

6. **Boost Your Metabolism** – plays a vital role in health and weight management. An active metabolism helps burn stored energy at faster rates.

7. **Stay On Track** – Diet should be designed to be flexible. So You can diet for a few days when you are not able to follow a diet. It also provides you with strategies to get back on track if you've strayed from your plan.

8. **Exercise** – Do basic yoga and breathing exercises to a minimum 6 days a week or walk for at least 6 km a day or do stretches 2 3 segments depending on your physical fitness and capacity.

9. **Relax and Sleep** – Meditation, Yoga, hobbies, and 7 hours of sleep every night will refresh you mentally and physically and puts you in a positive frame of mind to achieve your health and weight goals.

10. **Record Your Progress** – You need to record your vital statistics, weight, and health status so as to check your

progress and take corrective actions when necessary to achieve goals.

Regular health check-ups are an important part of the program.

'D' factors –
Discipline, Devotion, Dedication, and Detoxification.

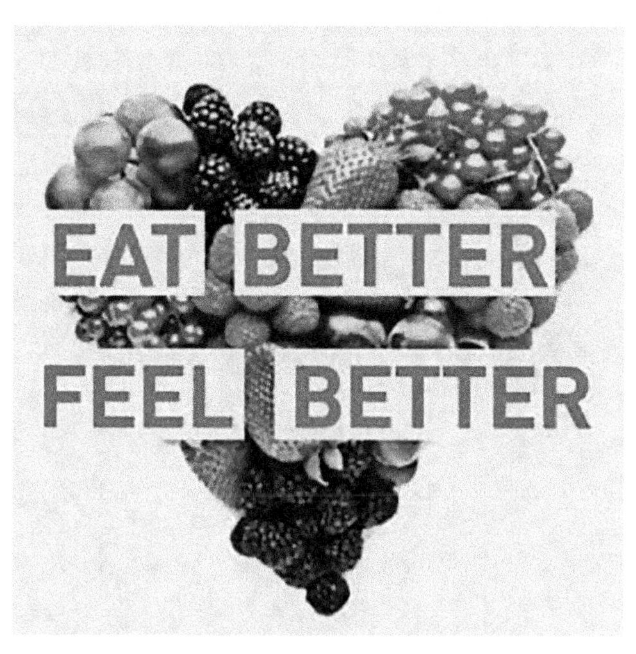

CHAPTER
Three

*Relearn — Your Relationship
with Food*

Comprehending Will Power

If we think of will power like a Red Carpet that admits only a selective few, we can't be more wrong. Will Power is like love, Compassion, or Wisdom. We all possess it. Everyone is invited and welcomed.

Will Power is a skill, to be strengthened and honed. You have to keep practicing it. With every 'No' you say to junk food, it becomes easier to say 'No', the next time. The more you affirm to those oily "Pakoras", the harder it will be to refuse them, the next time. It is as simple as that. Habits start off as thoughts in our minds. These thoughts set off a chain reaction within our body, leading us to act on the thoughts. But what leads to the translation and conversion of those thoughts into actions? That task can be accredited to the nerve cells residing in our body called neurons.

From the moment you thinking of devouring your favourite food, to the moment when you physically pick it up and eat it, the chain of Neurons works towards the translation of your thought into action.

This Chain is formally known and termed as "Neurons pathway".

Your brain has been wired to generate habits all the time, whether good or bad. The brain is likely to make habits because habits are sort of "Automatic" behaviour.

In the presence of Automatic behaviour, the brain is more inclined towards focusing on complex functions. And when you repeat a behaviour frequently, it becomes a part of your Personality.

Hence, the basic rule of building will power is to say "No" over and over again.

Closing the door on the old "You" is a little hard, in the beginning. When you are in the safety of your home, eating only nutritious and nourishing food, with all the junk tucked away and locked, it's a sign that you've built a strong will power. The test of your will power is when your friend comes over with pizza and coke. One of the two "You" will win the battle of will power then,

Old You: Maybe I can have a bite.

New You: Thanks, but I don't feel like eating it right now. Maybe, next time.

Boost Your Will Power

Eat Right and Eat more frequently. When you're eating all the right things, eating small portions at small intervals, there is sustained release of energy in your body, stabilizing your sugar levels. But on the other hand, if you wait too long before eating anything, or consume foods that are quickly converted to sugar, for instance, cakes and pastries, it spikes up your sugar levels.

That leaves you feeling tired, sluggish, and craving for more sugar. You then tend to eat more which weakens your ability to resist unhealthy foods for your next meal. It is a vicious cycle.

Love and Value Yourself

That Mirror on the wall is your best and most honest friend. Regardless of what people tell you, a mirror never lies. If you wish to change your body's shape, examine yourself in the mirror. Your Self-image or the mental portrait that you paint is more honest or distorted than any image reflected in the mirror.

It is no hidden information that the way you see yourself affects your behaviour and attitude towards yourself and others. Your emotions are also guided by your self-image and self-worth. How people perceive you, is often a reflection of how you see yourself.

You Deserve You

"Love yourself first, and everything falls into line".

Most of us are so used to putting everyone else ahead of ourselves. Spouses, children, jobs, business, friends, money, even fame- that somewhere along the way we cease to think of ourselves as being important enough to nurture, care, heal, and pamper.

We always give our best parts to others, reserving very little for our own self. So much so, that we ignore diseases and problems like stress, anxiety, depression, high BP and many more, just because we cannot take out a moment for our own selves and the listen to the message that our heart, body and soul are conveying to us-" Value yourself because you deserve it and you're worth it, and more!"

Loving yourself equates to celebrating your strengths and positive attributes, along with forgiving your flaws, blemishes, and shortcomings. It also means accepting and learning to live and love those you cannot. Dress yourself up in a way that'll make you feel confident and happy, and the rest of everything will fall into place.

- Keep reminding yourself that you're unique.
- Celebrate every achievement, no matter big or small, in every sphere of activity.
- Enlist everything you love and adore about yourself, your strengths, abilities, and talents.
- Stop comparing yourself with others.
- Pamper yourself- Treat yourself to regular massages, engage in a holiday, every once in a while.
- Forgive yourself- forgive your faults and failures, embrace yourself, be kind, and forgiving.

Your Body Image Is Important Part of Your Self Image

How you think and feel about your physical attributes is a reflection of your self-image. It is a commonly felt thought that there is always some room for improvement. Remember that perfection lies in the eyes of the beholder. Pick health over beauty every time and find natural ways to look and feel fresh, happy, and confident.

- Accept that there is no exchange, no return policy where your body is concerned. You have only one body, just this one form. So, make the most of it.
- Start from the top of your body, your head, your crown, and list down everything you love about yourself, your eyes, nose, the texture of your skin, shape of your

hands, etc.

- Work on enhancing and bringing out your best features. Dress yourself up in accordance with your body type and size.
- Write down things about your body that you'd like to work on.
- In the end, list the improvements which are in your control and only require diet control and a few changes in your lifestyle.
- Start making those changes and celebrate each advance towards improving your body image.

Your Diet

What you eat, the quantity of your intake, the frequency and nutritive values of the food you choose to consume, and your lifestyle, which may be sedentary or active has an impact on your weight. The better your metabolism and the more energy you burn through activity, the less your body weight, and vice-versa.

In other words, keeping all other physiological and external factors aside, you are solely responsible for your weight and body image, and only you can make a difference and begin to live a healthy life.

Miracles Do Happen

I am a strong believer in this statement. I have seen so many impossible and daunting looking tasks made possible by true efforts and sense of responsibility. As I said earlier, you are fully and utterly responsible for your own body. Nobody else is.

We always tend to make lame excuses to save our skin. My son was 125kgs in the year 2016 and now he is 90 kg. He lost approximately 40 kg just by strong will power and motivation. I always keep an eye on him, what he eats, his timings, water intake, balanced nutrition, etc. If he can do it, you can too.

Miracles do happen, be a part of them.

Measure Your Body

I always tell my clients, on the very first day, to measure a few things and jot them down.

- Chest
- Waist
- Mid-section around your navel
- Hips
- Thighs

Now, according to the International Diabetes Foundation, if a woman's waist size is measured to be more than 80 cms or 31.5 inches, or in case of men if it exceeds 90 cms or 35 inches, he/she is medically at risk of being unhealthy and have excess belly fat.

Measure How Tall are you

Measuring your height is really straightforward actually. Just stand tall with your back against the wall. Have someone place a ruler on the top of your head so that it touches the wall and mark the spot. Now, measure from that point downwards and note your height in cms or in inches.

Check Your Weight

Most of us only weigh ourselves when we're at the doctor's clinic. But its high time that we invest in digital or electronic weighing scales. Both of them are accurate and a breeze easy to read. The best time to weigh yourself is in the morning, after your ablutions, with very light clothes on.

Consult a Doctor

Don't forget to get your complete health check-up done, every once in a few months. The reports may uncover problems that should be treated before you start with your diet. Share all your concerns with your doctor. Some basic tests I recommend are:

- Blood Pressure
- Routine Blood and Urine tests
- Blood Sugar levels
- Lipid Profile–cholesterol and triglycerides
- Thyroid function tests

Get your tests done, twice a year from a reputed hospital and it will help you keep tab on your health. These regular check-ups will help you keep your lifestyle on track and warn if anything is amiss. They may not seem so important, but you'll see their worth, trust me!

FAT is not FIT

Is there anything wrong with being fat, overweight, or obese? You look larger than your size and your appearance may not be as captivating as it could be. You lose your self-confidence. Excess weight makes you lethargic, lazy and it prevents you from leading an active life. All in all, those extra pounds restrict your movement, slow you down, and make you physically unfit. Not to say that being overweight puts you in the direct path of some very serious life-threatening ailments.

- **Diabetes**

  A lifestyle-related disease caused by stress, irregular eating habits, lack of physical activity and a diet loaded with fat and sugar.

- **Heart Diseases**

  Your heart is unable to cope up with the excess body weight and so it builds up fats within arteries that carry blood to the heart.

- **Hypertension**

  The "Silent Killer", as everyone calls it, is directly related to obesity and a sedentary lifestyle. Excess body fat and salt in your diet increase the pressure with which your heart needs to pump out the blood, leading to hypertension.

- **High Cholesterol**

  The human body produces two types of Cholesterol: the LDL or bad cholesterol, an excess of which leads to fat deposits within arteries. The other is HDL or good cholesterol, which is responsible for cleaning the bloodstream of excess fat, carrying it back to the liver for disposal.

  Excess body weight is known to contribute to an excess of LDL or bad cholesterol.

All Fat is not bad

Our society places much importance on being thin. Seeing models in that perfect hour-glass figure, women get depressed and start imagining themselves in size-zero figures. Beauty often rests in the eyes of the beholder. What we do is we embark on restrictive diets or start starving ourselves to achieve our weight goals. But that can lead to Vitamin deficiencies, anaemia, osteoporosis, eating disorders, or anorexic (total aversion of foods).

So, if we have decided to eat healthily and adapt a healthy lifestyle, we need to keep a keen eye on quality, quantity, and frequency of what we eat and drink. We all should bear in mind that all fat is not bad. A body without fat would be like a delicate, temperature-sensitive piece of equipment without the protective packaging. Fats form a protective layer around your vital organs like the liver, kidney, and heart.

Like a blanket, it provides excellent insulation against changes in external temperature, thus regulating the body temperature. Fat plays the role of a battery, storing up the excessive energy for when your body needs it. If you consume more starch or sugar than is the requirement, the rest is converted to fat.

Mindful Eating

'Eat Less, Taste More'
Mindful eating is the act of eating with thoughtfulness and Pleasure. The focus is on choosing the right foods,

enjoying your meal to the fullest, and leaving each meal with a sense of satisfaction.

Following are some habits to cultivate mindful eating:

- Eat your meals at regular times every day. Your body will get attuned to the rhythm, you will rarely feel the urge to binge or overeat.
- Eat at the table – not in a hurry.

Take some time out, to sit peacefully and eat, whilst you enjoy the taste of the food you eat. Take a break from all else and concentrate on your food.

- Relish Your Food – Enjoy every bit, savor the taste of each spoonful. Don't gulp the juices, sip them down slowly.
- Eat Slowly – Chew your food well. Digestion begins in your mouth only. Besides, your brain needs 20 minutes to receive the signal that you're full and satisfied.
- Eat small portions and eat till you are satisfied, not till you are full.
- Balance is essential. Make sure you have all the nutrients on your plate for complete benefits.
- Eat fresh and natural food – always eat healthy options. Avoid packaged and processed foods as they are full of additives and preservatives.
- Double the Pleasure – Eat with a friend or your family. Meals are more relaxing and enjoyable when shared with someone you love.

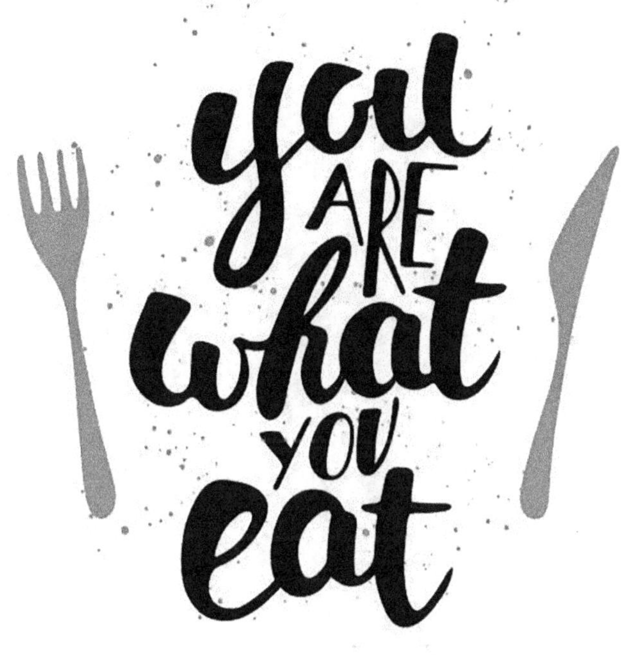

CHAPTER

Four

It's True, You are what you eat

Eat Sensibly

You may think that it does not matter what you eat. Well, it does. If you eat anything you want, it will show on your body. We all are food-centred ad everything we do revolves around food. Our closest relationships are formed by and nurtured through food.

Food memories are amongst the strongest memories we have. Memories invoked by food can whisk you back in an instant to a special time and place. I can never forget the tasty Thai noodles I ate at Phuket last year, the street side. The whole scene comes in front of my eyes. Flat Thai noodles, the man who was making them, my family waiting for a plate of noodles, and how we all were hogging Thai vegetables and noodles.

Flavour comes to my mouth even now when I think about that moment. So we relish our favourite foods, some relish golgappas, samosas and as soon as we name the dish, the flavours come to our mouth and we start relishing those moments, without realizing what we are doing right now.

Food nourishes and fills us with energy. It heals, cleanses, and fortifies. It soothes, comforts, and satisfies. But it can also hurt and harm, depress, and destroy. It all depends on what role you choose for it to play in your life. People in different countries eat differently. Each country consumes a certain amount of fats, proteins, and carbohydrates. None of us were created to eat refined and processed foods. Our bodies thrive best on local, organic, and fresh foods.

If we look back at Indian culture, we will notice that heart diseases, diabetes, and many other diseases were not rampant until refined and processed foods came to our market with adopting western culture. Now, we realize why the food we eat matters. In fact, your life and body size depends upon it. So always keep in mind, you are what you eat. And you will realize how your body responds to the food you feed it.

Let us talk about various food components and how they affect our health.

1. Proteins

The main function of the protein in our body is to promote growth, repair, and maintenance. Proteins are of special importance as they take longer to digest, give us the feeling of satiety much longer than foods that are rich in fats and carbs.

I see a lot of people on high protein diets gulping up to three protein shakes a day, and they are not even bodybuilders. Anything in excess is bad for your health. Excess protein that does not get utilized by the body is converted to fat. It puts a load on your kidneys. So we need to check protein intake. A normal human needs 0.8-1gm protein per kilo of your body weight. If you are 60kg, you need 60gm of protein in a day. Such a quantity can be easily obtained by a balanced Indian diet.

If you think you'll become thin by consuming more protein, then you need to check on carbohydrates and fat ratio too. Your body is the best indicator of your health. And deficiency, if any. You'll listen to it. If you are deficient in protein you'll feel tired when you should not be. You will feel weak when you exercise. You'll get injured quickly and will take long to recover. You'll have hair fall issues and your skin will not be healthy.

Lack of protein weakens the body and damages the nervous system, whereas extra protein produces toxins, acids and can damage the liver, kidneys, and digestive system.

There are nine amino acids. A complete protein comprises of all nine. Eggs, meat, fish are good quality protein. Rajma and brown rice is complete and high-quality protein food. Dal and chawal are a great combination that contains all nine amino acids required by the body.

Foods that boost our protein levels are:
- Nuts(Almonds, walnuts, peanuts, and cashew nuts)
- Flaxseeds, sesame, sunflower, and pumpkin seeds.
- Green peas, spinach, green leafy vegetables.
- Soybeans, beans, gram, moong.
- Whole grains(wheat, bajra, ragi, amaranth)
- Milk and dairy products, paneer, tofu.
- Brown rice
- Mushrooms
- Dal
- Yogurt

- Meat and Poultry
- Seafood – fish and Sea fish

2. Fats

Fats are essential for building your body tissues and cells and helps in the absorption of some vitamins (A and D) in our body.

I remember my mom would always encourage me to eat nuts and homemade pinnis (laddoos), which made me angry at that time. Laddoos, dry fruits, chips, and samosa all contain fat but there is a huge difference in these fats – Good fat and bad fat.

Good fats are essential fats that are required for healthy brain functioning, a strong immune system, and maintain the body's hormonal balance. And its energy production. Bad fats are those which clog our arteries and cause internal inflammation. We need to choose the right kind of fat and consume it in the right way. Fats are broadly classified as –

1. Unsaturated fats (Good fats)
2. Saturated Fats (Bad fats)
3. Trans Fats (Bad fats)

a. Unsaturated Fats

These are called good fats because they can improve blood cholesterol levels, besides, they play many other beneficial roles. They are found largely in foods from plants, such as vegetable oils, nuts, and seeds.

There are two types of unsaturated fat.

Monounsaturated fats (MUFA)

Found in olive oil, peanut oil, canola oil, almonds, and sesame seeds.

Polyunsaturated fats (PUFA)

Found in sunflower oil, corn oil, soybean oil, walnuts, flaxseeds, and fish.

Omega3

These are an important type of polyunsaturated fat, the body cannot make them, so they must come from food. They are believed to reduce the risk of heart diseases and boost the immune system. They are found in fish and fish oil such as cod liver oil.

b. Saturated fats

Bad fats contain triglycerides. They raise LDL (bad cholesterol) levels. Foods that include red meat, full-fat dairy products, such as cheese, milk, ice-cream, butter, coconut oil, palm oil, chocolates. Saturated fats remain solid at room temperature.

- They build up in arteries causing them to narrow, a condition called atherosclerosis, and can lead to major heart problems.
- They tend to clump together and form deposits in the body, along with protein and cholesterol, get lodged in blood cells and organs, leading to obesity, heart diseases, and cancer.

- They increase the acetate fragments in the body, which in turn leads to an increase in the production of cholesterol.

c. Trans Fats (The Ugly Fats)

These are actually unsaturated fats that are made synthetically by the process of hydrogenation, turning liquid oils into solid fats. Trans Fats such as vanaspati ghee and non-dairy cream are used in processed foods to prolong their shelf life and in cooked foods, such as cakes, biscuits, pizzas, ice-cream, and commercial deep-fried foods.

3. Carbohydrates

These are the main sources of fuel for your body. They are broken down in the digestive system and enter the bloodstream as glucose. Excess glucose is stored in the form of glycogen in the liver and in limited quantity in the muscles. The great Indian diet includes some of the most nutritious carbohydrates to maintain a fast metabolism, we need a balanced diet that comprises of all the macronutrients–carbs, proteins and good fats.

The absence of good carbs, proteins, and good fats. The absence of good carbs can cause sleep disorders along with low energy and fatigue. Some healthy Indian Carbs are –

- Brown rice–Unmilled, unpolished brown rice is extremely nutritious. It is a great source of selenium, magnesium, manganese, and tryptophan.
Rice is easily digestible food, polishing of rice destroys

70% of all its vitamin B, chromium, zinc, fibre, and essential fatty acids. Rice is gluten-free.

- Wheat – Wheat is rich in fibre and tryptophan. Wheat bran is a bulk laxative and helps with regular bowel movement. Whole wheat is rich in Vit E, which is essential for healthy skin and hair. Whole wheat is true anti-cancer food. Wheat contains gluten which some people are allergic to. Gluten is found in oats, barley, and rye. Women who eat more wheat have their oestrogen levels in control. This is important because an excess of oestrogen gives rise to fibroids, breast cancer, and cysts.

- Barley – It is an extremely healthy grain and a great source of fibre and selenium. Due to high fibre content, barley has a low glycaemic index and recommended for people with diabetes. It can keep you feeling full for a long time, so great food to weight loss.

- Corns – It Contains folic acid, which helps lower homocysteine that causes damage to arteries. Corn is a rich source of Vit B1, B5, and C as well as phosphorus and manganese.

- Millets – Rich in fibre, protein, manganese, and magnesium this grain keeps you full for a long time and decreases the total inhale of calories.

- Oats – These are excellent in weight-loss and heart-friendly. They are rich in manganese, selenium, fibre, vitamins, and proteins. Consuming oats regularly is great for enhancing immunity. They are rich in anti-oxidants, keep the heart and arteries healthy.

4. Fibre

Bulk up your diet, eat more fibre. Dietary fibre-found mainly in fruits, vegetables, whole grains, and legumes is the best known for its ability to prevent constipation. Foods rich in fibre are healthy and help in maintaining healthy weights and lower the risk of diabetes, heart diseases, and some types of cancer.

What are Dietary fibres?

Dietary fibre is known as roughage or bulk, includes parts of plant foods you can't digest or absorb. Fibre is not digested by the body. Instead, it passes relatively intact through your stomach, small intestine, colon, and out of your body. It is commonly classified as soluble and insoluble fibres.

Soluble fibres

This type of fibre dissolves in water to form a gel-like material. It lowers body cholesterol levels and glucose levels. Soluble fibre is founded in oats, peas, beans, apple, citrus fruits, carrot, barley, and psyllium husks.

Insoluble fibres

This type promotes the movement of material through your digestive system and increases stool bulk. Whole wheat, whole brans, nuts, beans, and vegetables such as cauliflower, green beans, and potatoes are good sources of insoluble fibre.

The benefit of a high-fibre diet

- Lower cholesterol levels.
- Help control blood sugar levels.
- Aids in achieving a healthy weight.
- Helps you live longer
- Helps maintain bowel health

Daily fibre Recommendations

	Age of 50 years	Age 51 or older
Men	38 gm.	30 gm.
Women	25 gm.	21 gm.

Refined foods such as canned fruits and vegetables, pulp-free juices, white bread, pasta are low in fibre. The grain refining process removes the outer (C bran) from the grain which lowers the fibre content.

Another way to get more fibres is to eat foods such as cereals, granola bars, yogurt, and ice-creams with fibre added.

5. Minerals and Vitamins

These are essential nutrients that our body needs to work properly. We get all the Vitamins and minerals we need by eating a healthy and balanced diet.

Vitamins are divided into two groups:

- Fat-soluble and Water soluble
- Fat Soluble Vitamins

Fat Soluble Vitamins are found in animal products and foods that contain fat, like milk, butter, vegetable, oil, egg, liver, and oily fish. We don't need to eat foods containing fat-soluble vitamins every day because our body can store them. Vitamins A, D, E, and K are fat soluble vitamins.

- Water soluble Vitamins

They come from fruits, vegetables, milk, dairy, and grains. They can be destroyed by heat or exposure to air. They can be lost in the water while cooking, especially when boiling food. Steaming or grilling, use the cooking water to add flavours to soups and stews are good ways to preserve water-soluble vitamins. Water soluble vitamins include vitamins C and vitamins B1, B2, B3, B6, B9, and B12.

- Minerals

Minerals are found in foods like cereals, bread, meat, fish, milk, dairy, nuts, fruits, and vegetables. We need more of some minerals than others. As we need more calcium, phosphorus, magnesium, sodium, potassium, and chloride than we do iron, zinc, iodine, selenium, and copper.

Restrict your intake of salt to not more than 2gm or approximately 1 teaspoon per day. Remember all foods contain some amounts of salt or sodium naturally so add a pinch of salt to your food. Beware of hidden salt in packaged foods such as biscuits, sauces, ketchup, pickles, soups, noodles, papad, and namkeen.

It is hard to control salt while eating out, but you can avoid pickles, papad, extra grated cheese on top of pasta, or chutney.

Food heals and protects

"Let food be thy medicine else medicine be thy food". Apart from providing us important nutrients, food is the ultimate healer for fighting diseases, food is the best cure, the best regulator of the body's health, and the best medicine. It is right that food can cause harm to your body if taken in excess or in the wrong proportions.

The secret is to eat more foods that are beneficial to health and avoid the ones that harm your body.

Antioxidants

These are the compounds that inhibit oxidation. Antioxidants are vitamins and minerals and enzymes that help to counteract the negative effects of oxidation of the cells in the body. Harmful molecules called the free radicals produced within the body as the result of oxidation, damage to the body cells and may lead to ailments such as heart disease, cancer, arthritis, and strokes.

Foods which are rich in antioxidants are:

- Vegetables: Cabbage, cauliflower, broccoli, spring onions, bottle gourd, green leafy vegetables.
- Fruits: Apple. Pineapple, Papaya, Guava, Strawberry, Tomato, Amla, Citrus fruits like Orange and Lemon

- Herbs and Spices: Mint, Coriander, Basil, Parsley, Chilies, Cinnamon, Cloves, Turmeric, Ginger.
- Nuts and Seeds: Almonds, Walnuts, Flax seeds, and Sunflower seeds
- Fish, Olive oil, and Green tea.

Food Cleanses and detoxifies

As a part of the digestive and metabolic processes, our bodies produce toxins that need to be expelled regularly and efficiently. So that the body can function well in an optimum way. Water is the main detoxifying agent in our diets. Drinking plenty of water allows the body to flush out toxins from the system. Detoxification has direct effect on BMR, helping to increase it and promote weight loss. To detoxify our body:

- Eliminate or restrict alcohol, smoking, refined sugar, Trans fats, and other harmful foods that act as toxins in our body.
- Eat plenty of fibre, whole grain, fresh fruits, and vegetables.
- Drink beverages that have detoxifying effects as lime water, vegetable juices, and green tea.
- Drink at least 3 4 litres of water every day.
- Pranayama or deep breathing exercises cleanse your system by allowing oxygen to circulate more freely.
- Exercise ramps up your metabolism and tones up your body so that they work to cleanse the body effectively.

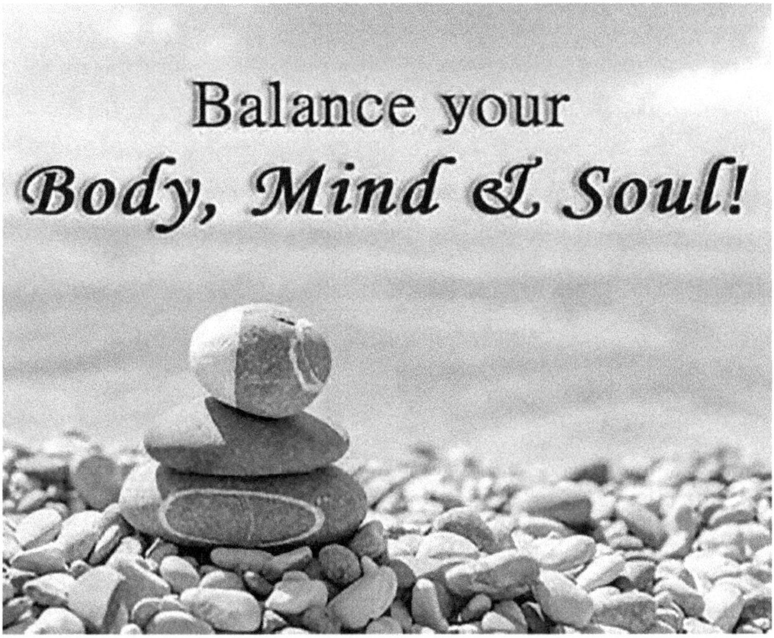

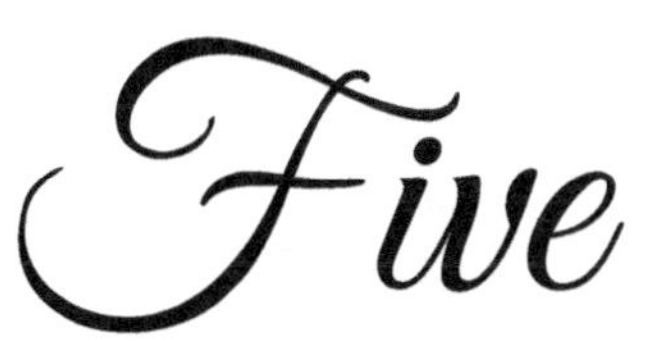

CHAPTER

Five

Healthy Body, Mind, and Soul

One of my clients who is a doctor says he had irregular working hours, so he ate without thinking of his health. However, he knew that in his profession he needed to be energetic, and healthy. My Programme focuses on yourself and to discipline your life. He says he is happy to meet me and my diet provides proper nutrition to him. He feels happy, healthy and his skin glows. His metabolism is so active now, he burns what he eats. He exercises regularly and has no excessive weight now.

He had tried many yo-yo diets earlier but had not succeeded in maintaining his weight or appearance. But Diet Well weight loss program with the combination of diet and exercise helped him reduce weight and maintain it.

Drink to your Health

Drink natural beverages that provide you with nutrients, fibre, hydrate your body, and activate your metabolism, and help to detoxify your system.

Detoxifying Vegetable juices

Raw, uncooked vegetables are a natural way of detoxifying the system as well as providing the body with essential nutrients. Raw vegetables preserve all the nutrients that are destroyed while cooking. Vegetable juice is particularly beneficial at the start of the day as it contains natural fibre which will kick start your digestion and helps evacuate your bowels. It also metabolizes fatty tissues, which is essential for weight loss.

Bottle gourd juice

The bottle guard is packed with hefty nutrition and a healing punch. Make sure you use tender, seedless bottle gourd. It is diuretic which helps to eliminate extra water from your body and prevents indigestion and acidity.

Green Tea

It has a soothing and calming effect and various health benefits, especially weight loss. Squeeze lemons into it and it becomes more beneficial. Green tea contains antioxidants that prevent damage to the body cells. It also prevents oxidation of bad cholesterol (LDL) and promotes the production of good cholesterol (HDL) and is an appetite suppressant.

Wheat Grass Juice

It is nothing but tender shoots of the wheat plant. It is very easy to grow at home in tiny pots in a warm, sunny place. Sow wheat grains in soil and sprinkle lightly with water every day. Tender shoots of wheatgrass will start to emerge and by the 7th or 8th day will be ready to have. Use only the top part of the grass. Wash it well, grind it, and then strain it to make a nutritious drink.

Wheatgrass juice has many health benefits. It contains beneficial enzymes, lowers blood pressure, purifies the blood, and increases red blood cells.

Carrot Beetroot juice

These two wonder vegetables are responsible for increasing your blood flow, reducing blood pressure, detoxifying blood, and keeping health problems at the bay due to the presence of antioxidants and nutrients. It helps in detoxifying due to the help of betaine in beetroot that helps to support healthy liver function. Carrot helps to excrete toxins from the body effectively. Take 1 carrot, ¼ beetroot, and 1 glass of water and blend them. Don't sieve the juice, take with the pulp for better benefits. You can add rock salt, lemon, and cumin powder to it to enhance the flavour of the juice.

Lime Water

Lime water helps to lose weight naturally and helps your body to improve its immunity and digestion. It is antioxidant, reduces skin pigmentation, skin hair fall, and delays greying of hair and make your skin glow. It also reduces leg cramps and improves blood circulation.

Aloe Vera Juice

Aloe Vera is a succulent plant that is used to improve skin and hair and cures skin care problems including burns. It is also a healthy food supplement with many positive effects on the body. It improves digestion, has detoxifying effects, and promotes healthy skin. It has a mood-lifting and soothing effect which is a good antidote to stress.

Coconut water

It is a refreshing, natural nutrient booster. It is rich in minerals and vitamins and low in fats. It is an excellent way of hydrating the system without any adverse effects. It is rich in potassium, it prevents cramps, and it helps in weight loss too.

Buttermilk

North Indians' favourite drink in the summers. It is perfect for a weight loss diet as it is rich in calcium and protein while low in fat. The good bacteria and enzymes present in it have a pro-biotic effect which aids in digestion and boosts the immune system.

Spices for Your Health

1. Cinnamon (dalcheeni)

We have seen that consuming as less as half a teaspoon cinnamon per day reduces blood sugar, bad cholesterol, and triglycerides in diabetic patients. Cinnamon can sweeten your life without causing diabetes. This spice with a peculiar taste has super inflammatory powers and helps in reducing arthritic pain. My experience is that if you have cinnamon powder and black peppercorns after your meals, it cuts down sweet cravings to a great extent and helps in digesting the food. Cinnamon is a good spice.

2. Turmeric (Haldi)

It is a fresh underground stem, dry them in bright sunlight, and powder them to store for a whole year.

Turmeric is bright yellow in colour and due to the presence of powerful polyphenol, cur cumin, imports various health benefits. It has the ability to fight cancer and neurodegenerative diseases. Its anti-bacterial and anti-fungal properties make it very beneficial when it comes to common health problems like cold, cough, and sore throat. It has great antiseptic properties also.

3. Fennel (Saunf)

It is filled with phytonutrients and antioxidants. A tomato fennel soup with garlic and a fresh salad with fennel bulbs makes it ideal for elaborate course meal. Plain roasted fennel is good for digestion.

4. Cumin (Jeera)

It aids digestion which is probably why we like chewing cumin seeds at the end of every meal. It has more health benefits beyond digestion too. Add cumin to your bread, fried beans, and sauce and a dish rich in flavour and high in health! We even love to add cumin in our regular bowl of dal tadka and rice too.

5. Oregano

It is used on pizza and pasta topping, oregano proves its worth as a potential agent against prostate cancer.

6. Heeng (Asafoetida)

It is widely used in Indian cooking. It has a strong pungent aroma. It is highly recommended for people with indigestion, stomach upsets, bloating, and intestinal gas.

You can add ½ teaspoon of heeng to water or buttermilk to get instant relief in case of digestive problems.

7. Green Cardamom (Elaichi)

It is the most aromatic of all Indian Spices. It is consumed in two forms – Choti elaichi (Green Cardamom) and Badi elaichi (Black Pods). Bad breath, loss of appetite, depression, indigestion, nausea, etc., cardamom cures it all.

8. Cloves (laung)

These dried flower buds of the clove tree are considered one of the 'hottest' among the spices. It has anti-bacterial and anti-septic properties. It is used as a remedy for toothaches for ages.

9. Black Peppers (Kaali Mirch)

It is a fruit of the black pepper plant. It has a pungent taste. It helps to relieve symptoms of the common cold. It can add black pepper to your hot vegetable soup and enjoy it when you have a cold.

10. Fenugreek (Methi daana)

Methi seeds are tiny, light brown in colour, and are better to taste. They are used in particular recipes like kadhi as well as various curries. Methi seeds can be soaked overnight and consumed early morning to stabilize your blood sugar, cholesterol levels, and flush out toxic elements from the body.

11. Legumes (dal, faliyan)

These are the plants that produce pods with seeds. They are classified with the following types:

- Lentils: 'Dal' is a common name of lentils, red lentils, brown lentils, and black lentils.
- Beans: Beans are neither a fruit nor a vegetable but a seed that is used as a food to eat. Kidney beans, moth beans, and soya beans are some of the most commonly used beans.
- Peas are green seeds that are eaten as vegetables.
- Peanuts develop in pods which ripen underground.

Legumes are a good source of carbs, protein, fibre, and low in fat. They are packed with calcium, iron, magnesium, potassium, and zinc. They are easy to cook and store.

For vegetarians, lentils are a good source of protein and help them build-up muscle to get a lean and toned body.

12. Salt (Namak)

Salt is an indispensable ingredient in all cooked food. It imparts flavour to food and is also used as a preservative. Sodium binds with chlorine to form sodium chloride known as table salt. We need to limit our sodium intake to not more than 2300mg salt per day. We can easily get the required amount from food. There are three kinds of salt available in the market.

a) Sea salt (Samudri Namak)

This is made after evaporating ocean salt and includes very little processing. It ensures the salt retains most of the nutrients.

b) Rock Salt (Kaala Namak)

It is the mineral form of sodium chloride.

c) Table Salt

It is the most processed form of salt from which most of the nutrients have been washed away.

13. Saffron (Kesar)

Kashmir is known for the product of the best quality in India. This ingredient adds colour and spice to biryani or dessert. Saffron is expensive but the benefits are priceless

Saffron has the ability to treat depression, prevents loss of vision, and improves memory. The stigma of flower can relieve you from the digestive issues with the help of anti-inflammatory, antioxidant, and anti-depressant properties.

14. Nutmeg (Jaifal)

Like clove, nutmeg has anti-bacterial properties. It helps fight tooth decay. Nutmeg can fight Alzheimer's and improve your memory. It can also release the tension in your muscles.

15. Ginger (Adrak)

It has been used to help digestion, reduce nausea, and help fight the flu and common cold.

16. Mustard (Sarson)

This seed comes from the ground and has a spicy flavour. Mustard helps reduce pain, stimulates appetite, and relieves symptoms of arthritis. Include mustard oil to your regular diet for benefits to your heart health. It keeps a check on blood fat levels and helps in circulation.

17. Sesame (Til)

This seed has a nutty taste. It has cholesterol-lowering compounds. It helps in balancing hormones and boosts nutrients absorption. Sesame seeds are rich in Vitamin B and iron.

10 Tips for Healthy Mind Body and Soul

1. Make the choice to put your health first

If you think this is selfish then you're wrong. You need to dig deeper and discover your soul is your inner being. If we can't control ourselves than how can we take care of the others. Choose wisely while eating. It is for your own good. Healthy eating will give you a peaceful feeling in your soul as well as a positive effect on your body. You need to believe in yourself.

2. Do things that you love

It gives you the opportunity to get in touch with your soul. The way we treat our bodies is a reflection of your own selves. The better we treat our bodies the better we are to ourselves. Find healthy food to eat and you will see how better you feel. Your energy levels will boost up and sleeping patterns will be better.

3. Establish a relationship with your body

We all have different shapes and sizes but the way we carry ourselves through everyday life sends a message to the world. Taking care of your body and well-being makes you feel good about yourself which in turn makes you feel better about other things in the world. Your little changes in diet add up to big results about feeling better about yourself.

4. Take part in Nature

Nature truly is great for our well-being and psyche. Time spent in nature has numerous benefits on our physical, mental, social, and psychological well-being and emotions. Going out in nature will improve focus, concentration, enhance your energy, reduces depression, improve happiness, and physical health. Feed yourselves with fruits and vegetables. It is a healthy dose of fibre which leads to good digestion and your body gets essential vitamins and minerals.

5. Let Go and Release

Exercise enables us to be free from all other issues for some time. Exercise is a stress reliever and enables us to think more clearly about our lives and God. We are able to release many emotions, thoughts, and feelings.

6. Find an exercise you enjoy

Whatever form of exercise you choose will make you happier. We get strong physically and mentally too. Exercise is key to healthy body and soul. Even half an hour's walk with your friends and partner will give you numerous health benefits. So don't skin your exercise routine.

7. Build Confidence and self-esteem

Always feel confident about yourself. Self-love is the first love. Building confidence and self-esteem are in our control. Find a sensible diet plan that works for you and boost your self-confidence. Seeing your body transform over the weeks and feeling healthier each day will improve your confidence and self-esteem.

8. Try Meditation

Meditation clears your mind and promotes awareness. A calm mind equals a calm soul. Everything is created within you. Including a healthy body and a mind. Take out some time to practice mindfulness. Feeding your soul, honouring your body, mind, and spirit will provide you a healthy mind and a healthy body.

9. Keep A Journal

Expressing yourself on a blank paper helps clarify your emotions, remove stress and solve problems in a calm and creative way. Expressing yourself in a journal is good for the soul. Write down your food choices too. Those who write down what they eat are more likely to have success in weight loss programs.

10. Do Away your doubts

Enhance your soul and take away the fear of failure. Ditch your anxiety about making the wrong decisions.

Throw out your self-doubt. Once you do it, you'll be able to make a difference in your well-being and the rest of the world. You are capable of much more than you think. I am a live example of this. I was a simple housewife taking care of my kids and family. Once, I realized my self-worth, I am done. See the changes in me.

Eating in a healthy manner will ensure that you are in control and can take charge in changing your body and well-being.

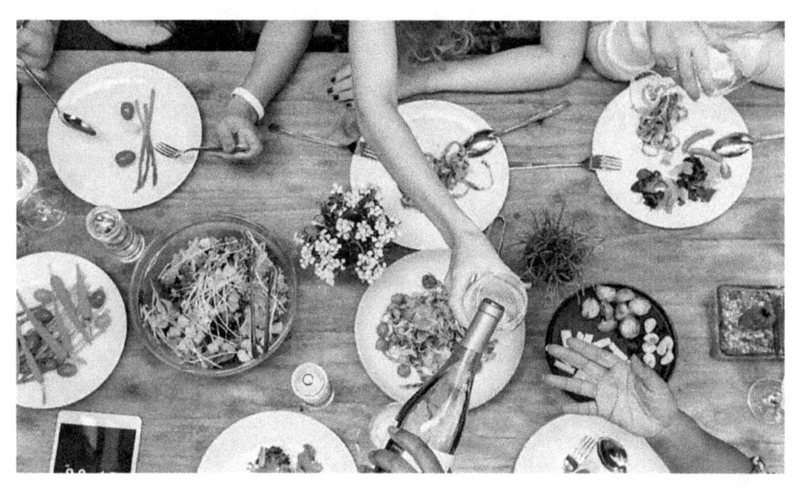

CHAPTER

Six

Manage Eating Out (Dining Out)

We all enjoy eating out and go to restaurants and coffee shops. Many clients of mine are fond of eating out twice a week. So you need to discipline yourself when you go out and check your eating habits. The biggest problem is when you eat is

1. Increased Temptation
2. Large portions
3. Intake of refined foods, fats, refined, sugar, and salt.

You need to plan before having joyful experience and keep weight loss goals. Here are a few tips to try while eating out:

1. **Read the menu before you go:** If you're not familiar with the menu, read it before you go to the restaurant. The sight and the smell of food when you are hungry can make it difficult for you to choose the right foods.

2. **Have a healthy snack before you arrive:** if you're hungry when you arrive at a restaurant, you may end up eating too much. One way to prevent this is to eat a healthy snack before you get there. A low calorie, huge protein snack like Yogurt could make you feel fuller and prevent overeating.

3. **Drink Water Before your meals:** Water is a fantastic choice for drinking before meals instead of sugar-sweetened drinks. Replace your mocktails (sugar-laden) with water and reduce the intake of calories and added sugar. People who drink 500ml water half an

hour before a meal, eat fewer calories, and lose more weight than those who don't drink water.

4. **Check how food is cooked and prepared:** The way the food is cooked has a significant impact on the number of calories it contains. Choose the foods that are steamed, grilled, roasted, or poached. Foods that are described on the menu as par-fried, crisply, crunchy contain more fat and more calories.

5. **Try eating your meal mindful:** Mindful eating means the conscious choice about what consumes and gives full attention to its eating process. Mindful eating helps healthier food choices in restaurants. It also helps to improve your self-control and prevent overeating.

6. **Order your meal before everyone else:** if you are eating with a group you are likely to order something that doesn't fit into your healthy eating plan. So make sure you order first, keeping your health into consideration.

7. **Order two appetizers instead of a main:** You are more likely to overeat when you're served with bigger portions. In restaurants where you know portions are huge, try ordering two appetizers instead of the main course. By doing this, you tend to eat fewer calories.

8. **Slow down and chew thoroughly:** Chewing food thoroughly and eating food slowly could help you eat less. It will help you feel full more quickly. Next time when you're eating try to count the minimum number of chews per bite to stop yourself from eating too quickly. You need to chew a bite 28-32 times so that it

gets mixed with saliva properly in our mouth and the process of digestion starts there and then only.

9. **Have a cup of coffee instead of a desert:** Skip dessert and order a cup of coffee instead. It will cut down your calorie intake and you will get some great health benefits associated with coffee.

10. **Avoid all you can eat buffets:** When you are at a buffet table, there is an unlimited supply of food, eating the right amount of calories can be challenging. Try using a small plate to help you eat less. If you take a normal-sized plate, fill half of the plate with salad and vegetables, avoid any kind of gravy and deserts at a buffet.

11. **Ask to make a healthy swap:** Most of the people tend to eat fewer vegetables. Vegetables are great as they have very few calories but lots of fibre and nutrients. For example, broccoli and spinach are extremely low on calories, but high in Fibre, Vit C, and all sorts of beneficial plant compounds. Increasing vegetable intake can reduce the risk of many ailments like cancer, obesity, and depression. When you order food, ask the waiter to swap a part of your food like fries with extra vegetables, salad, etc.

12. **Ask for sauces or dressings on the side:** Sauces and dressings can add a lot of calories to a dish, so ask for your sauces on the side. Instead of dressing laden salad, you can ask for dressing and salad separately, and it'll be much easier to control the number of calories you eat.

13. **Skip the pre-dinner bread basket:** Prefer to have a low carb diet at night. Avoid bread baskets, instead, opt for healthy options like green veggies, sautéed veggies, chicken (roasted or grilled), and salads.

14. **Order a soup or salad to start:** Having a bowl of soup before the meal can stop you from eating too much. It reduces total calorie intake by a total of 20%. Any soup or a plate of salad (without dressing) can be a healthy option.

15. **Share with someone else (or order half portion):** People who successfully lose weight have often shared food or ordered a half portion when eating out. It is the easiest way to cut back on calories and prevent overeating. If you have nobody to share with, you can pack the rest of the food for you to take it home with you.

16. **Avoid Sugar-sweetened and drinks:** Many of us have too much sugar in our drinks and it can be too much for us. Drinking sugar-sweetened drinks is strongly linked to an increased risk of obesity and type-2 diabetes. If you want to make a healthy drink choice while eating out, stick to water, and unsweetened green tea.

17. **Use Small measures of Alcohol:** Drinking alcohol can add a number of calories to your meal. The number of calories in the alcoholic drink varies depending on the strength of alcohol and the size of the drink.

18. **For instance, a large glass of red wine**, 1 cup (250ml), and alcohol by volume can add 280 calories to your meal. That's the same as a snickers chocolate bar. If you want to enjoy the drinks, cut back on the calories by

ordering smaller measures such as a small glass of wine.

19. **Go for Tomato-based sauces instead of the creamy ones:** Choose tomato or vegetable-based sauces instead of cheese or creamy ones to cut back calories and fats from your meal.

20. **Watch out for health claims:** Dietary labels can find their way into the restaurant menus. You may see a food highlighted as 'paleo', 'gluten-free' or 'sugar-free'. These labels don't mean that your choice is healthy. Added sugar and fats can be hidden in those foods to help them taste better.

21. **Think about your whole diet:** There are times when you eat your favourite meals for pleasure without thinking whether they are healthy or not. Being flexible about your diet is directly linked to better overall health and weight management. If you are feeling healthy meal patterns most of the time, then you can treat yourself occasionally. Indulgence can be good for the soul.

Diet Soda, Good or Bad?

Diet sodas are popular beverages all over the world, especially among people who want to reduce their sugar or calorie intake. Instead of sugar, artificial sweetness such as aspartame, saccharin, or sucralose is used to sweeten them. Almost every sugar-sweetened beverage has a 'light' or 'diet' version. Diet coke, Zero coke, Pepsi max, spirit zero, etc.

Despite being free of sugar and calories, the health effect of diet drinks and artificial sweetness is controversial.

Diet Soda isn't nutritious

Diet soda is a mixture of carbonated water, artificial or natural sweetness, colours, flavours, and other food additives. It usually has very few or no calories and no significant nutrition. For example, diet coke contains no calories, no sugar, or protein and 40mg of sodium.

Diet soda may improve fatty liver and does not appear to increase heart-burn or risk of cancer. It may reduce blood sugar and increase the risk of depression, osteoporosis, and tooth decay.

So if you are looking to decay regular soda in your diet, other options may be better than diet soda. Try milk, coffee, black or herbal tea, green tea, or fruit-infused water for weight-loss and I am sure you're going to get amazing results.

Tips to Control weight For North Indians:

1. Avoid curries. The gravy has the most fat. If dining out, take pieces of chicken or paneer out of the gravy.
2. Choose Tandoori foods.
3. Avoid dal makhani and other creamy gravy items. Ask for yellow dal without tadka or jeera daal for healthier options.
4. Avoid paranthas, pooris, and pulao. Opt for tandoori chapatti or steamed rice.
5. Whole wheat tandoori roti is preferable to bread made of refined flours like naans (butter or garlic).
6. Avoid khoya based or deep-fried desserts.

Tips for South Indian foods:

1. Idlis and dosas are high glycaemic index foods. Try to keep them within your grain allowance. One large idli or dosa (without masala), plain dosa.
2. Avoid potato-based masala in dosa.
3. Dal vadas well-drained and squeezed is a good choice.
4. Dahi vadas with rasam, Sāmbhar with vegetables are good fillers.
5. For non-vegetarians, chicken or fish with vegetables is a good option.
6. Keep away from heavy gravies and desserts.

Tips for Chinese Food:

1. Start your meal with soup, preferably without corn flour.
2. Go easy on fried appetizers, steamed dim sums is a better option.
3. Order steamed rice instead of fried rice, check the portion of rice and noodles.
4. Remember the half-plate rule. Fill up at least half of the plate with vegetables.
5. Lightly stir-fried vegetables, tofu, chicken, and fish are good choices.
6. Steamed fish with vegetables is a good option to eat out.
7. Beware of sweet and sour dishes as they are better coated and deep-fried.

Tips for Italian Food:

1. Skip bread or breadsticks. Ask for salad and olives instead.
2. Choose grilled seafood, lean meats, or breast of chicken with vegetables.
3. Ask for more vegetables in your pasta.
4. Choose thin-crust pizzas over regular pizzas. Two slices of a pizza are filling enough.
5. The white creamy mushroom sauce tends to be high on fats or calories. Try a tomato-based sauce instead.
6. Add a dash of parmesan cheese or olive oil to the dish – they add to taste and make you feel satisfied.

Tips for Lebanese food:

1. Go for falafel, chicken kebabs, or fish with salads.
2. Restrict Pita bread and wraps.
3. Avoid heavy desserts like baklava.

Tips while traveling, meeting, conferences:

1. Plan your day and reserve most of your food intake for social engagements.
2. Avoid heavy dinners. If unavoidable skip chapatti, naan, sweets.
3. Balance out your diet the next day.
4. Don't forget to have a cup of green tea after the main meal to digest it.
5. Eat healthy during meetings, avoid unhealthy snacking on biscuits and fried foods.
6. If possible keep lunch light.

7. Conferences offer food with rich buffets, eat wisely.
8. Watch your alcohol intake.
9. While traveling, carry healthy snacks like nuts, sweets, and fruits to avoid unhealthy eating.
10. Try to stick to your exercise regimen as far as possible.

Holidays and Manage eating (Vacations):

Vacations are meant to recharge you. People overindulge in food and drinks and go off their exercise schedules. They not only gain weight but it makes them feel sluggish and tired.

1. Be Active: Exercise regularly. Continue to exercise during your holiday. Go for a walk, swim, and run, play a sport or cycle outdoors.
2. Choose one favourite meal for the day and choose other meals light, consisting of salad, vegetables, and soup. Be an alert eater in breakfast buffets.
3. If possible plan dinner at normal meal time so that it is digested easily before bedtime. Late-night large meals contribute to overeating.
4. Carry snacks like nuts, seeds, whole grains to munch on so that you don't buy and eat unhealthy snacks.
5. Watch your drinks. Count for alcohol calories.
6. Towards the end of your holiday, make a few dinners light. It will help you in balancing your diet.

Manage Your Sweet Cravings:

Most of us enjoy sweets and desserts. Some of us have a compulsive sweet tooth. Sugar is addictive: the more you have, the more you want it. So try to manage sweet cravings. You have to break the vicious cycle.

1. Limit refined carbohydrates
   Carb rich foods like white bread, pasta may not feel sweet but they are forms of sugar. Choose healthy and low glycaemic index carbs instead, like whole grain, barley, oats, pulses, fruits, and vegetables.
2. Sugar cravings are often a consequence of missing nutrients. These include protein, zinc, Vit B, magnesium, and good fats. So a handful of nuts or roasted grams might be a good thing to reach for when you are craving a chocolate cake.
3. Fresh fruits and dried fruits like raisins, apricots, figs and dates, etc. should be your preferred sweets.
4. 'Sugar-free' fixes include mouth fresheners like fennel, cardamom, and sugar-free gums. Avoid these.
5. Increase the intake of raw vegetables.
6. Drink lemon water, green tea, green coffee, herbal tree to control sugar cravings.
7. Try to assess how often you have sugar cravings during the day. If you find them very often, set a target that you'll fight them more than giving in to them.
8. Lose belly fat.
9. Exercise Regularly.
10. Try to walk for 5-10 minutes after having four meals and change the posture of your body while sitting after every hour. Have a walk in the room for a few minutes and then come back to your work mode on the laptop. This will help you fight deposits in your body.

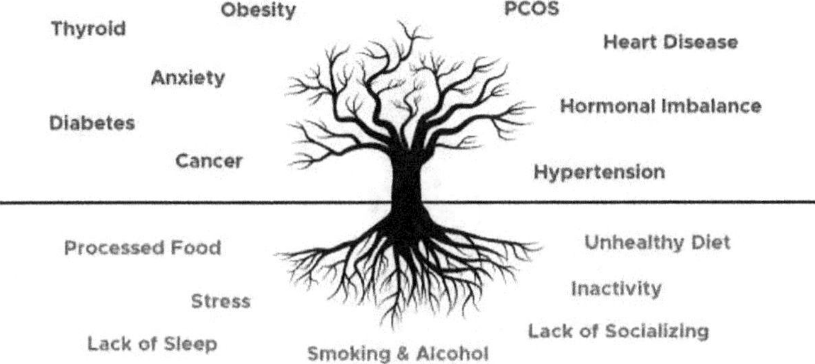

CHAPTER
Seven

Ageing and Lifestyle Diseases

Menopause – Coming of age-Natural Phenomenon

At around the age of 50, the ovaries stop producing oestrogens. The adrenal glands (small organs at the top of each kidney) continue to make oestrogens as does fat tissue. Our ovaries have produced the greatest share of the body's oestrogens for decades and when they quit, the blood levels of oestrogens drop quickly. Most women go through this change feeling fine, both physically and psychologically. Some women are bothered by the systems, including hot flashes, depression, irritability, anxiety, and other problems.

Menopause in many ways is like marriage, every woman has a unique one. How difficult or smooth your menopause will depend upon various factors, not the least of which is your nutritional status.

A woman who enjoys or feels in control of her body typically the one who has learned to take the responsibility of her well-being both physically and mentally. She is in tune with her body, mind, and senses that she has both intelligence and sensibility to understand that menopause is not a disease or a condition.

It is a natural phenomenon. What comes naturally to the body should not be feared or made a big deal out of it. It should only be understood and accepted (celebrated).

Nature to the Rescue

Nature has taken care of its female species, especially those of the human form because nature perceives it as special, intelligent, and important enough to be protected and nurtured and want us to go out of its way to allow us to thrive lead a fulfilling and meaningful life.

That is exactly why it created menopause for us. Nature has the wisdom to understand that a woman's energies are better directed towards care and nurturing her existing offspring so that it improves their fitness and survival, instead of directing them to produce more off springs that take a toll on her health and reduces chances of survival and good health of the younger ones.

Healthy Ovaries, Healthy Menopause

Our ovaries with age go through change and therefore the hormones change too. An Ovum is the largest cell in the human body. With time the size of ovaries starts decreasing. And so does the production of hormones. As long as you have ovaries, your menopause can be smooth. For that, you need to make sure your diet remains nutritionally rich and do exercises daily.

Regular exercising keeps the waist slim and prevents it from thickening. A thick waist makes you prone to a host of lifestyle diseases, weaker bones, joints, etc. the biggest danger than gaining weight around menopause is the change in fat distribution. The only sensible thing is to have an active and healthy lifestyle and allow hormones to go through their natural transition and maintain the balance.

A poor nutritional status makes smooth menopause impossible. Lack of exercise results in a lack of circulation and oxygenation to the ovaries, making it difficult to go through menopause.

Nature creates conditions for us to have smooth menopause. The problem is we don't support nature. Most women gain weight. They start following the yo-yo diets, weight loss plans, diets without consulting a dietician which destroys their nutritional balance especially Vitamin D, calcium, and b12.

If a woman works toward her menopause as nature does, it will not become a phase where you gain weight or prone to high blood pressure, heart diseases, vaginal dryness, osteoporosis, hot flashes, sleepless nights, etc but a natural, smooth and much-needed progression towards a healthier, meaningful and insightful existence.

Life after Menopause

Most of us lead lives limited by our hormones and menopause forces us to think beyond their limitations. Our periods have ceased but we still exist. Overcome your limitation and soar above all horizons you set for yourself. A lot of women feel angry and irritable around menopause, even the most gentle, caring, and loving women too.

The body creates a hormonal situation by wearing off progesterone and oestrogen, make it difficult for women to exist.

Women tend to feel irritable that they may have made mindless adjustments and compromises, may feel angry and depressed. There is nothing wrong with feeling irritable, angry, and depressed really. The insight one gains during menopause finally allow women to understand that living life on her terms and conditions doesn't mean she'll create havoc in someone else's life.

We need to have some kind of training that allows us to direct our anger, guilt, depression.

Writing down your niggling thoughts gives you a chance to understand yourself and fulfil your wishes. We need to channelize our efforts to be the person we want to be, it actually allows us to sleep well at night.

We need to realize all the stories of mood swings, irritability, and sleepless nights are just misinterpretations of nature's blessings.

Foods to Eat

There are certain foods that help to relieve some symptoms of menopause such as hot flashes, poor sleep, and low bone density.

Dairy Products

The decline in oestrogen levels during menopause can increase women's' risk of fracture. Dairy products such as milk, yogurt, and cheese contain calcium, phosphorus, potassium, magnesium, and vitamins D and K are essential for bone health. Women who eat animal protein have comparatively higher bone density than those who don't.

Healthy fats

Healthy fats such as omega3 fatty acids may benefit women going through menopause. Need to add supplements that decrease the frequency of hot flashes and night sweats. Foods high in omega 3 fatty acids include fatty fish and flax seeds, chia seeds, and hemp seeds.

Whole Grains

Whole grains are high in nutrients including fibre, vitamin B. A diet high in whole grains reduces the risk of heart diseases, cancer, and premature death.

People who eat 2 or 3 servings of whole grains have a 20-30% lower risk of developing heart diseases and diabetes. Whole grains include brown rice, whole wheat bread, barley, quinoa, etc.

Fruits and Vegetables

Fresh fruits and vegetables are packed with vitamins and minerals, fibre, and antioxidants. Women who eat more vegetables, fruits, and fibre, and say experience less hot flashes, and attribute to a healthy diet and weight loss.

Phytoestrogen- containing foods

Phytoestrogens are compounds in food that act as weak oestrogens in our bodies. Foods that naturally contain phytoestrogens include soybeans, chickpeas, peanuts, flaxseeds, grapes, berries, plum, green tea, and black tea.

Quality Protein

Women going through menopause should eat more protein. Foods high in protein are eggs, meat, fish, legumes, and dairy products.

Foods to Avoid

Avoiding certain foods may help reduce some symptoms linked to menopause such as hot flashes, weight gain, and poor sleep.

1. **Added Sugars and Processed Carbs**

    High blood sugar, insulin, resistance are linked to a higher incidence of hot flashes in menopausal women. Processed sugars and added sugars are known to raise blood sugar rapidly.

    So limit your intake of added sugar and processed food such as white bread, crackers, and baked goods.

2. **Alcohol and Caffeine**

    Caffeine and alcohol can target hot flashes in women going through menopause. Caffeine and alcohol are known to be sleep disrupters and women going through menopause have trouble sleeping. So avoid caffeine and alcohol near bedtime.

3. **Spicy Foods**

    Avoid spicy foods during menopause. Spicy food intake increases anxiety and hot flashes in menopausal women.

4. **High Salt foods**

    High salt intake is linked to lower bone density in postmenopausal women. After menopause, the decline in oestrogen increases your risk of developing high blood pressure. Reducing sodium intake may help lower this risk.

These simple changes in your diet may make an important transition in your life easier.

Thyroid (Hypothyroid)

The thyroid gland is butterfly-shaped and is in our neck in front of our windpipe. Its function is to produce a group of hormones, collectively called 'thyroid hormones'. The thyroid hormone regulates our body's metabolism and the way your body utilizes carbohydrates, fats, and protein for growth, development, and energy is every cell of the body and regulates the temperature of our body.

It also produces 'dopamine', the feel-good hormone. And it influences every other hormone in our body because everything in our body is interlinked. So if thyroid hormones don't work with efficiency, then all the other hormones like oestrogen, insulin, etc. suffer too.

Due to this imbalance, it takes a toll on our neurotransmitters and enzymes. And if they are feeling out of sync our vitamins and minerals synthesis is affected and in turn our metabolism, calcium absorption, sleeping patterns, mood stabilizers, alertness, everything suffers.

The main thyroid hormones are t4 and t3. Thyroxin or t4 is considered as the precursor to more active triiodothyronine or t3 and is present in many large amounts and has a larger half-life than t3 (that is it sustains itself longer in the body). The thyroid is controlled by the pituitary gland which is the size of a peanut and is located at the base of the brain. The pituitary gland produces the thyroid-stimulating hormone (TSH) which tells the thyroid gland to produce T4 and T3.

Now, once TSH is released, the thyroid needs iodine and tyrosine to produce t4 and t3. Iodine is involved in making thyroid hormones. Without adequate iodine, in your diet, you're fighting a losing battle against fat loss.

Tyrosine is the protein that iodine bonds with, to make thyroid hormone, is a nonessential amino acid whose levels in our body are controlled by essential amino acid L-phenylalanine. So an adequate intake of protein is required by our body.

So, to conclude

Tyrosine along with Iodine makes thyroid hormones=the normal function of thyroid hormones to optimize metabolism that works well=fat that burns well=Healthy well-being.

Thyroid and Weight Loss

Our body is interlinked as discussed before. So just one organ or hormone is not causing a problem to the entire body. We need to work hard on ourselves, adopting a healthy lifestyle, healthy eating, and exercise rather than being stressed about hormones.

Yes, the thyroid can have an effect on high triglycerides levels, diabetes, sleeplessness, painful periods, fatigue, low Vit D, and weight gain. We have to follow some strategies and play smart with our bodies:

Foods to eat:

There are plenty of options we have:

- Eggs, whole eggs are the best as Iodine and selenium are found in the yolk and egg-white is full of protein.
- Meat: All meats including lamb, chicken, fish, seafood.
- Vegetables: all vegetables are fine to eat in a moderate amount, especially when cooked.
- Fruits: All fruits including oranges, bananas, berries, tomatoes.
- Gluten-free grains and seeds: Rice, buckwheat, quinoa, flax seeds, and chia seeds.
- Dairy: All dairy products including milk, cheese, and yogurt.
- Beverages: water and other non-caffeinated beverages.

Foods to avoid

- Soy-based foods like tofu, beans, soy milk.
- Cruciferous vegetables: Uncooked broccoli, kale, spinach, cabbage, etc.
- Fruits like peaches, pears, and strawberries.
- Beverages like tea, coffee, green tea, and alcohol, as these may irritate your thyroid glands.

Tips to maintain a healthy Weight

It is easy to gain weight with hypothyroidism due to slow metabolism. Here are a few tips to maintain a healthy weight:

- Practice Mindful Eating: Pay attention to what you're eating, why you're eating, and how fast you're eating can help you develop a better relationship with food. It helps to lose weight food.

- Try Yoga and meditation: It can help to de-stress and improve your overall health.

- Get Plenty Of Rest: Aim to get 7-8 hours of sleep every night. Sleeping hours of sleep every night. Sleeping less than this is liked to weight gain.

- Try at a low moderate carb diet: Eating a low to moderate amount of carbs is very effective for maintaining a healthy weight.

So we can conclude that thyroid friendly diet can minimize your symptoms and help you maintain a healthy weight. It encourages eating whole, unprocessed foods, and lean protein.

PCOD/PCOS

PCOD (Polycystic Ovary Disease) and PCOS (Polycystic Ovary Syndrome) are likely the same but different. PCOD means that your ovaries are reeling under pressure and feeling burnt of disturbances in your body and generally not working at their peak efficiency.

PCOS means that these disturbances are no longer just in the ovaries but also in the other parts of the body- as acne and body hair. Irregular period, obesity, insulin sensitivity, high amount of male hormones, high blood pressure, difficulty in conceiving, and oily skin. In PCOS, many small fluid-filled sacs grow inside the ovaries. The wold 'polycystic' means 'many cysts'.

These sacs are actually follicles each one containing an immature egg. The eggs never mature enough to trigger ovulation. PCOS affects up to 27% of the women during their childbearing years. It involves cysts in ovaries, high levels of male hormones, and irregular periods.

What causes PCOS?

Mainly high levels of main hormones prevent the ovaries from producing hormones and making eggs. Genes, insulin, resistance, and inflammation are all linked to excess androgen production.

Lifestyle issues are one of the reasons. Women are competing with men in all fields of life like managers, heads of business executives, etc. they get very little time to take care of their eating habits, and they don't have time to cook so they eat processed foods.

They have coffee for breakfast, grab lunch (pizza, burger, sandwich) available in the office and dinner is usually late (around 9:30-10 pm) they don't have time to exercise instead of crammed traffic conditions instead of walking – so inactive lifestyle. It increases the total bad fat percentage and your body weight increases.

Insulin resistance-up to 70% of women with PCOS have insulin resistance means their cells can't use the insulin properly. Insulin is a hormone that the pancreas produces to help the body, user sugar from foods for energy. When cells can't use insulin properly, the body's demand for insulin increases. The pancreas makes more insulin to compensate. Extra insulin triggers the ovaries to produce more male hormones.

Obesity is a major cause of insulin resistance. Both insulin and obesity can increase your risk for type2 diabetes.

Inflammation

Women with PCOS often have an increased level of inflammation in their bodies. Being overweight can also cause inflammation.

How to take care of your health

If you have effortless and regular periods, it shows your fitness levels (it means all hormones, enzymes, organs like ovaries, kidneys, liver, etc are keeping good health). Feeling comfortable during and before periods is normal. Felling uncomfortable, irritable, cramps during before or after periods are abnormal. It means your health is in poor shape. Start lowering your body fat levels and make it easier for your ovaries to breathe and please.

Lifestyle modification is a buzzword here. Information is the key.

Nutrition

Eat fresh, wholesome food, and low carb diets. A low glycaemic index (low GI) diet that gets most carbs from fruits, vegetables, and whole grains help regulate the menstrual cycle better than regular weight-loss diets.

Foods to Add In Diet

1. High fibre diet

These foods combat insulin resistance by slowing down digestion and reducing the impact of sugar on blood.

High fibre foods are:

- Cruciferous vegetables like broccoli, cauliflower, and sprouts.
- Green leafy vegetables
- Green and red peppers, sweet potato, pumpkin.
- Beans and lentils
- Almonds
- Berries

Lean protein sources like tofu, fish, and chicken don't provide fibre but are very filling and healthy dietary options for women with PCOS.

2. Anti-Inflammatory Foods

Foods that help reduce inflammation are beneficial. They include tomatoes, kale, spinach, almonds, walnuts, olive oil, and fatty fish high in omega3 fatty acids.

- Foods To Avoid
    * Foods that high in refined carbs such as white bread and muffins.
    * Sugary snacks and drinks.
    * Inflammatory foods such as processed and red meats. These include highly processed foods white

bread, breakfast pastries, sugary desserts, anything made with white flour.

Sugar is a carbohydrate and should be avoided wherever possible. Sugar is present in sodas and juices. It is a good idea to reduce inflammation-causing foods like fries, margarine, and processed food.

Diabetes

It is a condition that impairs the body's ability to process blood glucose known as blood sugar. Without ongoing careful management, diabetes can lead to a build-up of sugar in the blood, which can increase the risk of dangerous complications, including stroke and heart diseases.

Different kinds of diabetes can occur and manage the conditions depending on the type. Not all forms of diabetes stem from being an overweight or inactive lifestyle, some are present from childhood.

Three major types of diabetes are:

- Type 1 Diabetes: Also known as juvenile, this type of diabetes occurs when the body fails to produce insulin. People with type 1 diabetes and insulin-dependent, which means they must take artificial insulin daily to stay alive.

- Type 2 diabetes: It affects the way the body uses insulin while the body still makes insulin, unlike, is type 1, the cells in the body do not respond to it effectively. This is the most common type of diabetes as has strong links with obesity.

- Gestational diabetes: This type occurs in women during pregnancy when the body can become less sensitive to insulin. Gestational diabetes does not occur in all women and usually reduces after giving birth.
- Pre-diabetes: Some people have pre-diabetes or borderline diabetes when blood sugar is usually in the range of 100 to 125 mg/dl.

  Normal blood sugar levels sit between 70 and 99 mg/dl, whereas a person with diabetes will have fasting sugar higher than 126 mg/dl. The risks of pre-diabetes and type 2 diabetes are similar. They include:
- Being overweight
- Family history of diabetes
- History of high blood pressure
- History of PCOS
- Being more than 45 years of age.
- Have a sedentary lifestyle

Nutrition Strategies

- Don't skip carbs for dinner, you need that. Simply get wholesome ones instead of processed ones. Rice, Jowar, Bajra, Wheat, Barley, Ragi.
- Take care that you don't have low blood sugar levels. So, it is suggested to carry a packet of sugar or chocolate with you all the time.
- Selenium, zinc, chromium will help your insulin respond better. So ensure that your food is growing in soil and rich in nutrients.

- Without adequate protein, insulin will not function well. So eat complete meals. Like khichdi or kadhi + vegetable +curd or rice +dal + vegetables.

- Avoid high sugar foods that provide empty calories or calories that do not have other nutritional values, such as sweetened sodas, fried foods, and high sugar desserts.

- Engaging in at least 30 minutes exercise a day or at least 5 days a week such as walking, aerobics, cycling, and swimming.

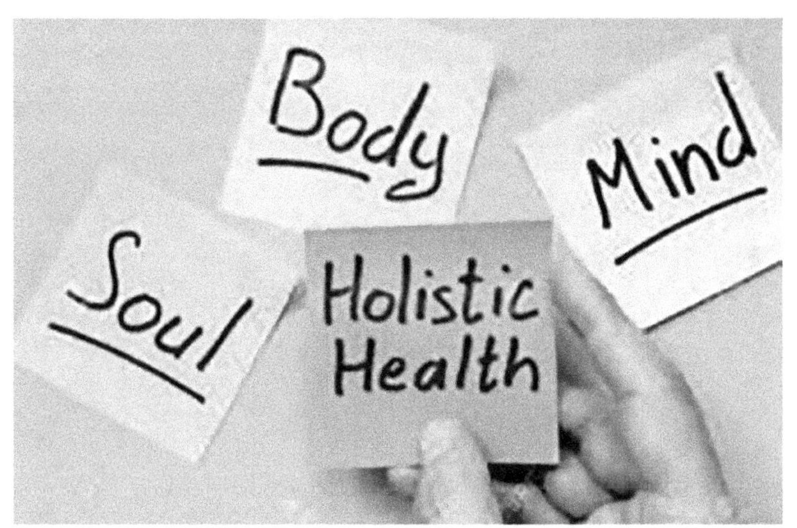

CHAPTER
Eight

Mental Health and Emotional Stability

Ways to reduce Mental Illness

Mental health includes emotional stability and maturity of character as well as the strength to withstand the stress of living without undue symptoms, physical or psychological. Mental and emotional health is not just the concern of those who suffer from it. Keeping mentally fit is as much of concern for everyone as is keeping physically fit.

Fight and not Flight from your problems. We're all problem solvers. We spend most of our lives on it. Therefore, we possess considerable experience in that. The first step is to understand the real nature of the difficulty. You may feel the need for help or counselling.

Get your facts clear, aim at accurate statements, keeping vagueness at bay, as it does nothing but causes unnecessary worry. Try to break down your problems to get at an easy solution. Ask relevant and frequent questions. The answers will help to define your problem. Become a relaxed and poised person.

Simplify your life – Simplifying refers to becoming aware of ways, big or small, that we expand money, time and energy, taking steps to curb the waste. The moment you decide to simplify your life and start putting in efforts for the same, you will find tolerance levels going up and everything around becoming less complicated and more beautiful.

Here are a few steps to gain control over life's hassles

in order to not have a stressful life and have time for pleasures:

- Start The Day Right

  Start your day half an hour early than your routine, by doing meditation. Prepare for the day in advance on the previous night. Always put the key in the same place, so that you don't end up losing them.

  Studies show that an average adult spends 16 hours a year searching for lost keys.

- De-Clutter Your Home

  Rid yourself from unnecessary possessions. Cultivating just one good habit can prevent the clutter from accumulating. Houses reflect not just a person's social status but also the owner's character, taste, and lifestyle. Overstuffing the house may obstruct physical movement and may not aesthetically appeal to the guests.

- Gently say 'No'

  'No' is a two-letter word that can free many hours a week. Say it gently but immediately (when the occasion requires so), offering a brief explanation. Try avoiding detailed excuses.

- Encourage Your Kid To Help

  Let kids know what is expected of them. They may know their duties like picking up their plates after they've finished their meals or picking and dropping the glass of water after drinking rather than playing all the time. They must know to share responsibilities with their parents.

Take Charge of Your Life

Here are four strategies which can turn adversity to advantage:

1. Assume responsibility for yourself: Time heals all wounds. It is important to deal with painful experiences. Some people cope by blaming God, fate, or others. But the truth is ultimately we have to assume responsibility for our own lives. Move beyond hurt and make something of your life.

2. Make Tough Choices: People who gain through experience feel it is not possible to go by avoiding risk and hoping all will turn out well. People grow because of the decision they make.

   Risks frequently pay large dividends. The ability to make a decision and act on it is a mark of good management.

3. Seek Relationships that enrich your life: Relationships are the web of life, they enrich how we think, feel, and behave. At times, they affect the course of our lives. Successful people often have friends or mentors who guide them during the early faces of their lives.

4. Affirm Self-worth: Typically, a crisis undermines one's self-esteem which makes it even more difficult to deal with the crisis. Those who are able to affirm a sense of self-worth are less likely to feel helpless and more likely to influence events and explore options when faced with adversity. We don't automatically incorporate good ideas into our lives, we grow by choosing to grow, by responding positively to what happens to us.

Outsmart Stress with Diet

It is the type of food you eat, not the number of calories that make a difference to your stress levels. Also, the amount of energy and fuel you need daily will vary.

There is a definite connection between the food you eat and the state of your mind. How?

Well, the amino acid called Tryptophan in starch activates serotonin. And when carbs are eaten with the Protein, the insulin released from the Pancreas prevents some other amino acids to enter the brain. This allows the tryptophan a clear field to work on, so it will give your mood a lift in just half an hour. Carbs are the body's main source of fuel. Unadulterated carbs may make you feel sleepy in a while. That is why it is essential to combine proteins with the carbs, cheese in your bread, meat/beans on your pasta, and dal with your rice.

Best carbs are beans that are a good protein source, brown bread, cereals, and grains (rice, barley, oats, wheat, millets), Rawa, pasta, vegetables (potatoes, sweet potato, pumpkins).

Six Vital Components of Food

1. Vitamins

   Used in numerous cell activities. Help to release energy from glucose and assist growth and repair mechanisms.

2. Minerals

   Sixteen different Minerals facilitating growth and repair mechanisms, help to release energy from nutrients, and help in forming new tissues.

3. Fibre

   Helps in the absorption of energy, producing nutrients, and helps in the digestion of food.

4. Carbohydrates

   Sugars and starches are broken down to provide energy. They are ideal foods to eat before exercise.

5. Fats

   Fats supply concentrated energy. They also help to form chemical messengers such as hormones.

6. Proteins

   Amino acids released from the digestion of proteins are used as building blocks in the formation of new cells. Good Nutrition is a term synonym with a healthy body. So we must balance between the quality and the quantity of the diet to sustain adequate nourishment. Generally, we think the primary concern of the food is just to satisfy our hunger. This misconception leads to improper selection of food choices.

Physical, Mental Illness during Covid-19 Pandemic

The Lockdown owing to the pandemic in our country was announced on 22nd march 2020. That led to huge changes in everyone's life. Some people got stuck in different cities and countries, distanced from their loved ones. They were not able to reach their homes. Some were not able to have access to food and daily basic requirements. People were confined to their homes only. From their daily busy schedules to business meetings, everything was disturbed and cancelled.

According to WHO, health is a state of complete physical, mental, and social well-being and not merely the absence of disease or infirmity

All the three steps of health were affected at some level in everyone's life in this lockdown. As India has different income groups, the problems differ accordingly. Furthermore, we're all at home, so chances are, no physical activity is carried out. But this immovability, doing nothing, just sitting in one place and eating has bad effects on one's health. The pandemic has also affected our incomes, which is the biggest cause of stress for all. Labourers and their families are suffering from a big-time financial crisis.

Physical and Mental health are related to each other in one way or the other. People are looking for counsellors and meditating apps to relieve their stress. Online appointments and meditating centres are doing good business these days. How to keep depression at the bay is everyone's main concern nowadays.

Now, we are to understand 'You are what you eat'. So eating clean and healthy food and exercising regularly has a very good impact on our mental health. Foods like Spinach, Cashew nuts, Chocolate, Cheese, walnuts, mushrooms, oats, avocados can help you in suppressing anxiety. Processed foods, junk foods, and sugar should be avoided if you're suffering from anxiety.

For physical health, walk around your house, you could opt for some stretching, yoga, meditation, etc. There are many home workout videos available on platforms like

YouTube. For mental health, you can do yoga, meditation, talk to a friend or video conferencing is a better option to see your loved ones face to face and talk to them. Thus all three aspects i.e. Physical, Mental, and Social Well-being are important in one's life and the absence of any one of them won't give peace but only transient happiness.

Fight Stress with Yoga

Yoga is more than just a bunch of simple routine exercises put together. Yoga helps in removing mental tension, fatigue, insomnia, and other ailments. It is the most powerful exercise that helps to remove and relieve stress, as well as relieve ailments which modern medicine has no cure for. Establishing a consistent yoga routine is the best way to experience the difference yoga can make.

Hatha yoga is the physical practice of yoga postures. There are different types of hath yoga. Some are slow and more focused on stretching, while the others are fast and more of a workout. If you're looking to relieve stress, no one yoga style is superior. So pick one that meets the level of your physical fitness and personality. Stretching relieves tension from the problem areas including hips and shoulders. Relief of low back pain is another benefit of yoga.

Breath Control

Pranayama is an important part of any yoga practice. Yoga increases your awareness of breath as a tool for relaxing the body. Just learn to take deep breaths and you'll realize that it can be a quick way to combat stressful situations and is amazingly effective.

Clearing the Mind

Our minds are constantly active. Racing from one content to another, spinning in full swing on incidents from the past. All this mind work is tiring and stressful. Yoga offers the technique to tame our monkey mind.

With each breath, you focus on the present moment, you are not breathing in the past on the future but only right now. Focusing on inhaling and exhaling. It clears the other thoughts from our minds.

These are basic meditation techniques.

Relaxation

Each yoga session ends up with five to ten minutes spent in relaxing in the corpse cope – Savasana. While this is enforced, relaxation can be difficult at first. Eventually, it serves the purpose of total release for both body and mind. Yoga Nidra is a practice that offers an opportunity for a longer, deeper period of relaxation and an introduction to meditation, which can be a great stress reducer.

Meditation

Meditation is not about becoming a new person or a better person or a different person. It is about training and awareness and getting a healthy sense of perspective. You are not trying to turn off your thoughts or feelings.

You are learning to observe them without judgment. And you may start to better understand them as well.

Mindfulness is an ability to be present, to rest in the here, and how fully engaged with whatever we are doing at the moment. It takes time to get comfortable with your mind. There might be setbacks on the way, but that is a part of meditating. Keep practicing.

Meditation may be used with the aim of reducing stress, anxiety, depression, and pain.

Maitri Bodh Parivaar

I joined Maitri Bodha Parivaar in 2019 January founded by our divine friend and love incarnate **"Dadashreeji"**. It is a family of friends bonded by a common mission to develop, nurture, and strengthen the human bond of love and friendship.

Maitri Bodh Parivar's work is aimed at transforming humanity through self-realization and preparing humanity to enter the new era of universal love and peace. Maitri Bodh Parivar's programs help reconnect with an individual's higher self. There begins the journey of inner awakening with direction, to fulfil the purpose of one's existence.

Vision

To establish love in everyone's heart through the human transformation with the help of true knowledge and divine intervention to attain one world, one community, and one truth.

Mission

Uplift human consciousness to a higher state where love, truth, and harmony will be the governing forces that will ensure the individual's transition to inner peace through our unique paths.

Values

- True Knowledge: Aatma Bodh
- Right conduct: Satya karma
- Selfless Service: Seva
- Bond with the Divine: Sambhandh
- Unconditional love: Prem
- Friendship: Maitri
- One Family: Ek Parivaar

Maitri Sambodh Dhyan

The purpose of this meditation is to communicate and connect to the higher consciousness and to bond with the divine. A guided meditation for the times, brought under the Grace and the guidance of **Dadashreeji**.

Maitri Sambodh dhyan is one of the most effective, easy to practice meditation processes, which helps us to connect with our inner being, the source, and our divine form. It establishes the bond and connection which is the most important and basic step to begin our inner journey of re-discovering our true nature.

I had great experiences in my life after practicing the process in the guidance of the divine friend **Dadashreeji.** It changed my life by 360 degrees, helping to involve a totally new me.

Thank you **Dadashreeji** for enlightening our lives.

The Power of Gratitude

The most powerful and inexpensive tool available on the planet is gratitude. Our minds dwell on problems not resolved, opportunities missed, relationships lost, promises not kept, poor health, and fears of an uncertain future, regrets, and longings. While life shares challenges and disappointments, it also brings us joy, problems solved, relationships built, great health, hope that reassures our fear, blessing upon blessing. It brings with it the opportunity to move forward even an inch each day, in spheres such as health, wealth, career, relationships, and spirituality. An opportunity to practice kindness and cut down on worry.

Gratitude is a thankful appreciation for what one receives, whether tangible or intangible. With gratitude, people acknowledge the good in their lives. People usually recognize that the source of that goodness lies at least partially outside themselves.

As a result, gratitude helps people connect to something larger than themselves, whether to other people, nature, or themselves.

We have seen the power of gratitude transform the health of extremely sick people. We see people throwing away their sleeping pills because they have understood that it was never the cure. The real cure lies in our minds. We have seen gratitude transform relationships and careers, and inspire people who would never work well or eat well, to start doing so.

Gratitude is strongly related to greater happiness. It helps you feel more positive, relish good experiences, improve your health, deals with all kinds of stress, and build strong relationships.

Tips to Cultivate gratitude in your life:

- Write a Thank you note: Write a thank you letter, expressing your enjoyment and appreciation of that person's impact in your life.
- Thank someone mentally: No time to write? Just think of someone who has done something nice for you, and mentally thank that individual.
- Count your Blessings: Pick a time every morning, before getting out of bed, to count your blessings. Identify them, be specific, and thank god.
- Pray: People who are religious can use prayer to cultivate gratitude.
- Meditate: Mindful meditation involves focusing on the present movement without judgment.
- Gratitude helps you refocus on what you have, instead of what you lack.

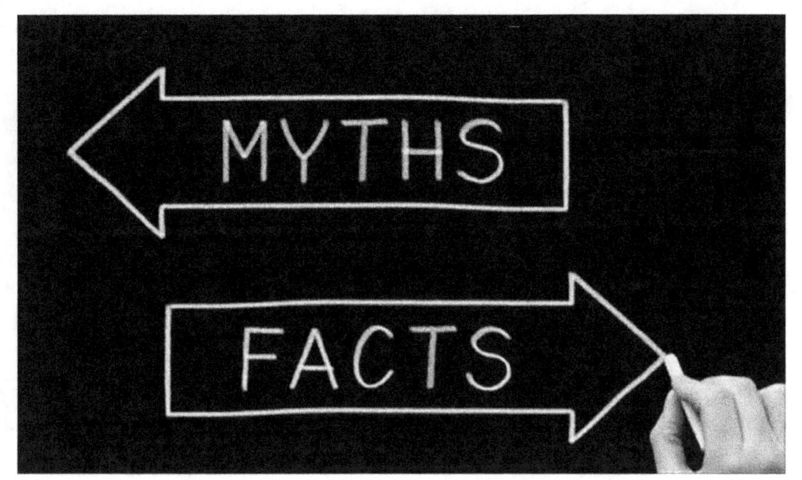

CHAPTER
Nine

Myths and Facts

1. **Myth: You should avoid all fat if you want to lose weight.**

   Fact: Fats provide essential nutrients and are an important part of the healthy eating plan. You need to limit fats to avoid eating calories. You can have healthy fats like avocados, olives, nuts, and avoid whole fat milk and cheese and have the low-fat versions.

   Use olive oil for cooking instead of butter.

2. **Myth: Dairy products are fattening and unhealthy**

   Fact: Dairy products are high in protein and our body needs them to build muscles and help other organs work well and the calcium strengthens our bones. Milk and yogurt are rich in vitamin D.

   Dairy products that are low-fat have few calories. Adults should have 3 servings a day of low-fat dairy products including milk, yogurt, cheese, or soy beverages.

3. **Myth: Going Vegetarian will help you lose weight**

   Fact: Going vegetarian, only will lead to weight loss is not the truth. We see Indian vegetarian diets are linked to lower levels of obesity, lower blood pressure, and reduces the risk of a heart attack.

   But you need to reduce the total number of calories. Some vegetarians make food choices that may lead to weight gains such as eating a lot of food high in sugar, fats, and calories.

Eating small amounts of lean meats can also lead to healthy weight loss.

4. **Myth: To lose weight you have to give up all your favourite foods.**

   Fact: You don't have to give up all your favourite foods when trying to lose weight. A small number of cheat meals could be a part of your weight loss plan. Just remember you must burn more calories than you put in for good weight loss.

   Limiting food high in calories may help you lose weight.

5. **Myth: Grains like bread, rice, pasta are fattening. You should avoid them when trying to lose weight.**

   Fact: Whole grains are healthier than refined grains. Whole grains include brown rice, whole wheat bread, cereal, and pasta. Whole grains provide iron, fibre, and other important nutrients.

6. **Myth: choosing foods that are gluten-free will help you eat healthily.**

   Fact: Gluten-free foods are not healthy if you don't have celiac disease. Gluten is a protein found in wheat, barley and rye grains. If you don't have any health issues, don't avoid gluten, you may not get enough vitamins, fibre, and minerals that you need.

   Gluten-free diet is not a weight-loss diet.

7. **Myth: Indian food is fattening and unhealthy**

   Fact: The excess of anything is bad for one's health. Overeating is known to store the extra food as fat in the body. Don't use extra oil, butter, sugar, or cream to enhance the taste of food. While cooking at home be mindful of things like the type, and the amount of oil used.

8. **Myth: Indian gravies are unhealthy**

   Fact: If gravies are cooked with lots of oil, cream, cashew nuts, and cheese in restaurants, they are unhealthy. My favourite gravies at home are based on onions, tomatoes, garlic, ginger, coconut, yogurt, besan, and garam masala made at home.

9. **Myth: Fruits can be consumed at any time in the day**

   Fact: Eat fruits only on an empty stomach, not after meals or with bread. Eat fresh fruits. Avoid packaged fruits and canned juices. If we consume fruits the right way and in the right quantity, first thing in the morning it has great benefits on health and skin.

10. **Myth: Skipping meals will help you lose weight.**

    Fact: When you skip a meal, your body's metabolism slows down to compensate for the lack of energy (food). Besides slower metabolism requires fewer calories. In addition, if you skip a meal, you tend to overeat at the next meal which results in more calories being consumed.

    For better appetite control, try eating this meal daily including small snacks between meals.

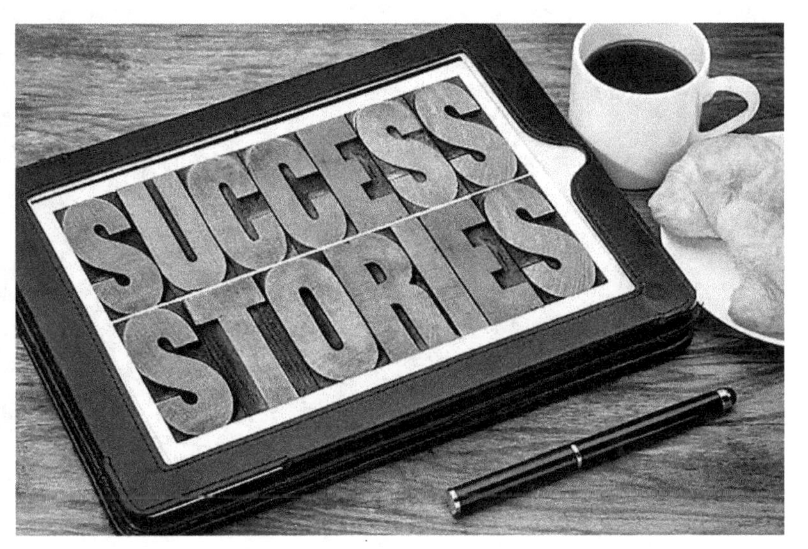

CHAPTER
Ten

Success Stories

Story 1

One of my clients, Rajesh (18 years, 5'10 height) had finished his school and was about to enter college life, was 120kgs when he came to me. Luckily he had parents who inspired him to have healthy eating habits, so they approached me in 2017.

He replaced his fast-food cravings with healthy home-cooked meals, eventually, he became more committed, changed his lifestyle, followed the routine of early dinner and early to bed (earlier he used to sleep at 4 am in the morning).

Now he goes to bed by 11 pm. In fact, losing weight and changing lifestyle was hard but he did it. Today he is 90kg and he says

'Give yourself a fair fight and take that blindfold off. It could propel you to places you never thought you could be.' Exercise and keep yourself hydrated all day.

He is following basic principles of life and maintaining his weight. Start his day with 1 fruit and eat frequently. Don't give long gaps between your meals.

Story 2

Reena, a 14-year old school going girl feels she is overweight and has tried so many diets in attempts to lose weight. She does not eat well because of the fear of putting more weight. Her mother is very unappreciative of her daughter's body and often nags her about it. No socializing and no recreational activities.

She even has really painful periods and a week before she starts feeling dull, sleepy, and lethargic.

I counselled her when she came to me. She had lots of things to do. School, tuitions, exercise, but no time to relax and eat nutritionally adequate food. At her age, she needed to have the right proportion of protein, carbs, fats, and other essential vitamins and nutrients.

Once her body had the right nutrients and she started exercising regularly, she started to lose weight and to love and appreciate her body and eating the right foods. She is happy now, her skin glows, her energy levels are much high and her body fat levels are dropped.

Today after 6 months, she is a totally transformed being.

Story 3

Simran, a 27-year old married mother of 2 kids. She has put on 20kgs weight after her marriage. Her younger daughter was 8 months old. She had to reduce her post-pregnancy weight. She had been suffering from sleepless nights and binge eating. She was looking for the right guidance

She came to me with her friend, my old client. She needed to change her eating habits and needed to change herself. She had lost her self-confidence and her body shape too. Then, after 2-3 sessions, her morale was boosted. She was mentally prepared to take responsibility for her body and her life.

Now, after 5 weeks of her diet, she has lost 7 Kgs, just by eating healthy, all kitchen homemade remedies. Today, she shared a picture with me showing she has 2-3 inches from her stomach and waist. She is more confident now. Ready to follow all my diet plans religiously. Her exercise routine is also going well.

So happy for MY HAPPY CLIENTS.

Story 4

When I started my practice 7 years ago, a middle-aged man (55-years old) came to me with 135kg weight, hypertension, alcohol consumption every day and dinner at night club every day.

Difficult client but I made changes in his eating habits during the day and only non-veg snacks (roasted food) at night with lots of salad and green vegetables. Increasing the water intake 12-14 glasses of water, 2-3 fruits in a day, mid-morning detox juices.

He followed the diet day long and at night only took snacks and salads. Then green tea before bed. Sunday was always a cheat day. Poori-bhaji every Sunday brunch. Slowly, I switched him to stuffed roti on Sunday but still, he loved Poori-bhaji every weekend.

After doing a diet for 6-7 months, he lost 30 kg and came to 105kg. Even today, he visits me or calls me up for advice and thanks me for healthy lifestyle changes he inculcated in his life.

Blessings for all the clients, God bless all with good health.

Story 5

A client of mine, 55-years old, hypertension, type 2 diabetes, depression for the past 5-7 years, post-menopause. Totally shattered. No way to go. Weight was ok, around 65kg. But she needed mental help.

I started counselling her and after 5-6 sessions of counselling, meditation, pranayama with me, 2 hours, 3 times a week, she started looking at the positive side of her life. I am a spiritual healer too, so she got spiritually healed. Her family history was that her mother died because of depression. She was so scared in her mind that one day she would also die like her mother.

But all thanks to the supreme power we helped to heal her and to come out for all her troubles. Today she is a healthy human with so many stories to tell to her children and her grandchildren. She laughs at her troubles.

I'm so happy for her. God bless her and spread happiness and love on this planet 'Earth'.

You have to totally surrender to god for your well-being.

My motto of life: 'I don't do - He does'

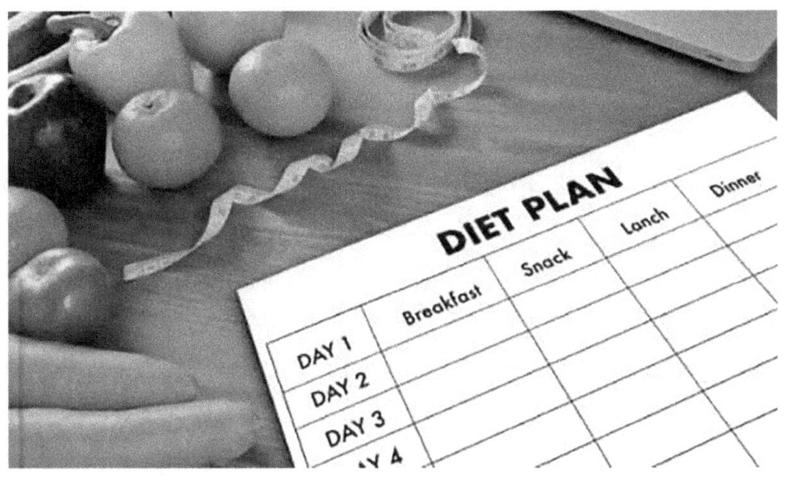

CHAPTER

Eleven

Sample Diets

FOR VEGETARIANS

- Early Morning – 2 Glasses lukewarm lemon water+5-7 curry leaves.
- After 1 hour – 1 fruit
- Breakfast — Veg sandwich (cucumber + tomato + mint chutney)
- Lunch – 2 chapattis+ green vegetables+ salad + curd
- After 1 hour–Green tea
- Evening – Tea/Coffee (without sugar) + a handful of roasted Makhanas
- Dinner – 1 chapatti+ Green vegetables + Salad
- Before bed – Turmeric Milk + Cinnamon

Important Tips:

1. Drink 10-12 Glasses of Water every day and 2-3 fruits Snack time.
2. Green Tea after Lunch and Dinner.
3. No fried food, no junk food, no Sweets.

Note: Diet has to be personally designed according to your lifestyle and eating habits. This diet represents you can eat everything, eat healthy and stay fit.

*I would like to design first free sample diet for you.

Please contact me at: soniakocharapp@gmail.com *

FOR NON-VEGETARIANS

- Early Morning – 2 glasses lukewarm lemon water
- After 1 hour – 1 fruit
- Breakfast – 2 egg whites + 1 slice brown bread +skimmed milk (1 glass)
- Mid-Morning – Orange/ Buttermilk
- Lunch– 2 chapattis+ Seasonal Vegetables/chicken curry+ Green Salad
- After an hour – Green tea
- Evening Snacks – Chicken Soup/Green coffee
- Dinner – Boiled Chicken/Roasted Chicken + Green Salad
- Bed Time – Toned Milk with Cinnamon and turmeric

Important Tips:

1. Drink 10-12 Glasses of Water every day and 2-3 fruits Snack time.
2. Green Tea after Lunch and Dinner.
3. No fried food, no junk food, no Sweets.

Note: Diet has to be personally designed according to your lifestyle and eating habits. This diet represents you can eat everything, eat healthy and stay fit.

I would like to design first free sample diet for you. Please contact me at: soniakocharapp@gmail.com

FOR VEGANS

➢ Early Morning – 2 glasses lukewarm lemon water

➢ After 1 hour – 1 fruit

➢ Breakfast – 2 pcs Banana Bread + hummus + Peanut butter

➢ Mid-Morning — Vegetable juice (with pulp)

➢ Lunch – 2 chapattis/brown rice+ Green vegetables+ Salad

➢ After an hour – Green tea

➢ Evening Snacks — Black tea/Green coffee

➢ Dinner-1 chapatti+ Green Vegetables/Sautéed Vegetables Green Salad

➢ Vegan person can have Almond milk, Soya milk or Coconut milk instead of cow/buffalo's milk.

Important Tips:

1. Drink 10-12 Glasses of Water every day and 2-3 fruits Snack time.

2. Green Tea after Lunch and Dinner.

3. No fried food, no junk food, no Sweets.

Note: Diet has to be personally designed according to your lifestyle and eating habits. This diet represents you can eat everything, eat healthy and stay fit.

I would like to design first free sample diet for you. Please contact me at: soniakocharapp@gmail.com

LET'S CONNECT

Facebook : https://www.facebook.com/dietwell/

Instagram : @dietwellbysoniakochar

LinkedIn : Sonia Kochar

Website : www.dietwellclinic.in

www.dietwellcoach.com

Email : soniakocharapp@gmail.com

Mobile : +91-9888112313

Sonia Kochar's Achievements

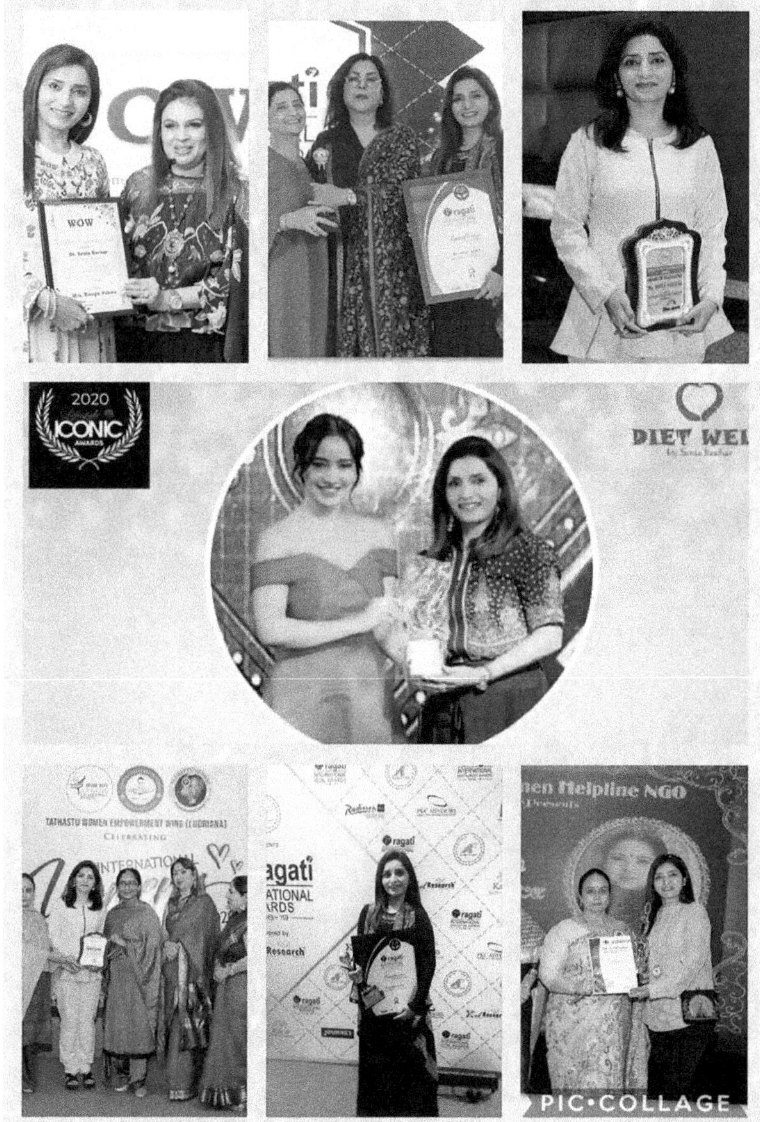

DietWell Health Awareness Club Activities

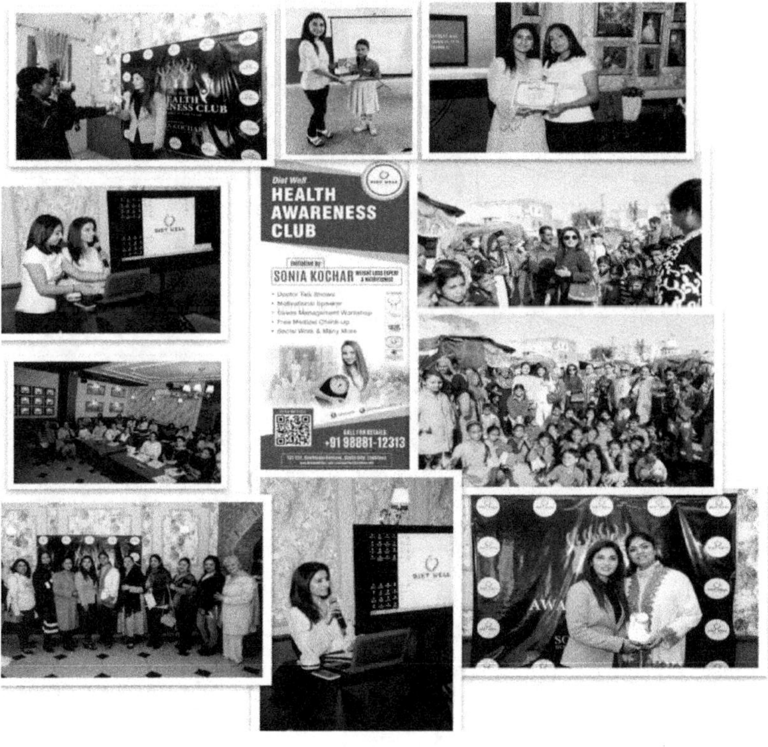

News Paper Articles

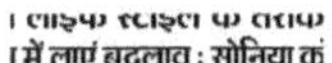

Get rid of weight this winter

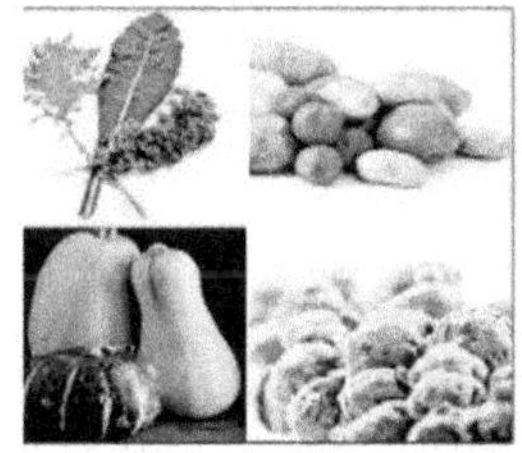

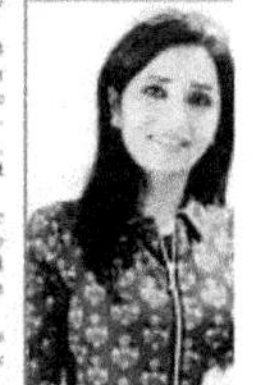

बाल भवन व सीनियर सिटि
होम में बांटे मास्क व सैनिटाइ

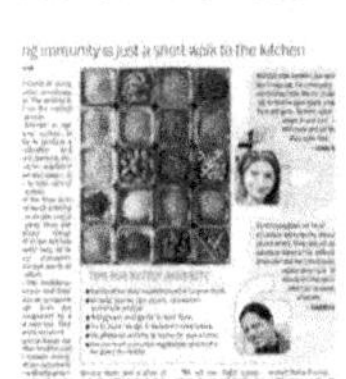

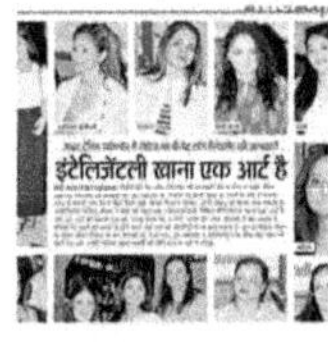

इंटेलिजेंटली खाना एक आर्ट है

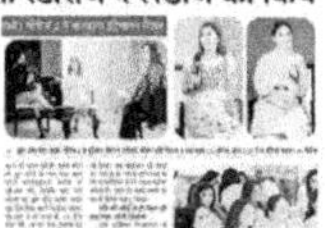

न रिच डाइट ज्यादा लें

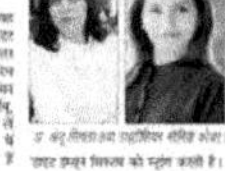

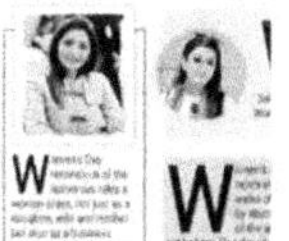

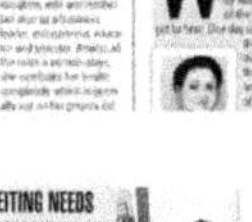

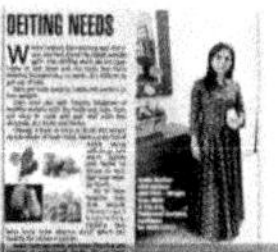

Winter season approaching and everyone worried about inevitable weight gain. Chilling short winter days make us rest more and our feel more relaxed. No excuse to walk... it's difficult to get out of bed.

Here are easy ways to follow this winters to lose weight:

Start your day with healthy instead of healthy cereals like dry fruits and nuts. They are easy to cook and pair well with few almonds, dry fruits every.

Have a bowl of soup or stew this winter as substitute to one meal. Have a plate full of salad along with soup. Add spices and herbs to soups to maintain your energy levels. Try to have healthy fats that

absorb important nutrients. Healthy fats help body soak vitamins A,D,E which are healthy for nervous system.

Avoid hydrogenated and trans fats that are present in processed foods. Try to have olives, olive oil, almonds, avocados, flaxseeds, walnuts, salmon in your daily diet regime.

Skip calorie laden Coffee and masala teas. Switch on to green tea and green Coffee and keep your body hydrated with drinking lots of water.

Savour sweets that slim you down. Avoid refined sugars and carbs. Have roasted beets, baked sweet potatoes and seasonal vegetables.

Avoid your comfort fried foods. Add fresh vegetables like cauliflower, broccoli, cabbage, carrots, spinach, peas, celery to your diet. Steam, bake or stir fry vegetables in little olive.

Munching time try to seasonal winter fruits. your day with 1 fruit. You have pomegranate, kiwi, apple, figs, grapes, pear, ora. Have different fruits thro out the day. You will lose weight very fast.

There are few winter weight loss tips that all should practice. You don't need to choose expensive foods to reduce weight. Even seasonal fruits and vegetables and simple kitchen remedies can help you lose weight. Don't fol fad diets but eat healthy and reduce weight this winter.

Sonia Kochar
Diet Advisor
DietWell - Weight Loss Diets
131-132, Sukhmani Enclave, Ludhiana
M: 9658112313